MEDICINE IN THE POSTWAR WORLD

The March of Medicine, 1947

NUMBER XII OF
THE NEW YORK ACADEMY OF MEDICINE
LECTURES TO THE LAITY

MEDICINE IN THE POSTWAR WORLD

The March of Medicine, 1947

The New York Academy of Medicine

Essay Index Reprint Series

Originally Published by
Columbia University Press
New York

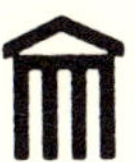

BOOKS FOR LIBRARIES PRESS

FREEPORT, NEW YORK

Essay Index

The Committee on Lectures to the Laity is composed of Clarence P. Oberndorf, M.D., Chairman, John M. McKinney, M.D., Arthur M. Master, M.D., representing the Committee on Medical Information; B. S. Oppenheimer, M.D., Ralph H. Boots, M.D., and Alexander T. Martin, M.D., representing the Committee on Medical Education; and Kirby Dwight, M.D., representing the Committee on Public Health Relations. Iago Galdston, M.D., is Executive Secretary.

Library of Congress Cataloging in Publication Data

New York Academy of Medicine.
    Medicine in the postwar world.
    (Its Lectures to the laity, no. 12. The march of
medicine, 1947) (Essay index reprint series)
    Includes bibliographical references.
    1. Medicine--Addresses, essays, lectures.
2. Psychiatry--Addresses, essays, lectures. I. Title.
II. Series: New York Academy of Medicine. Lectures
to the laity, no. 12. III. Series: New York Academy
of Medicine. The march of medicine, 1947.
R111.N435 1947   610   78-167392
ISBN 0-8369-2468-1

PRINTED IN THE UNITED STATES OF AMERICA
BY
NEW WORLD BOOK MANUFACTURING CO., INC.
HALLANDALE, FLORIDA 33009

FOREWORD

IT is appropriate that the twelfth series of Lectures to the Laity given in 1946–47 under the auspices of The New York Academy of Medicine should be devoted to Medicine in the Postwar World. During the fateful years through which the peoples of the world have recently passed, our populations have felt the stirring of great progress in the control of disease as the aftermath of the recent world-wide totalitarian war, and their desire for more knowledge of these momentous events in the field of the medical sciences is still unsatisfied. No one is better qualified to tell of these achievements than the Surgeon General of the Army.

It required little perspicacity to decide that the public needed more information on atomic energy and the revolutionary repercussions of this new field of research upon every clinical and laboratory branch of medical science. It was also not too difficult to select as another subject for popular presentation the so-called "antibiotic" drugs which are, curiously, derived from harmless molds in the air or bacteria in the soil, and which have an enormous but still unmeasurable value not only in the cure of infections of many kinds but, even more significantly, in preventing the spread of pathogenic bacteria from person to person. The application of atomic research to medicine and the employment of the antibiotic drugs for the control of the infectious diseases are unquestionably two most significant accomplishments of the war period which will bear rich fruit in future years and serve ultimately to compensate, at least in part, for the recent senseless destruction of human life and the spread of human misery.

In selecting the remaining three Lectures to the Laity, the Committee has departed from the traditional conception that the concern of the physician must be predominantly with physical ailments. In devoting three out of the six lectures to problems of psychiatry and of human behavior the Committee lays pointed emphasis upon the fact that by far the greatest lesson which the war has taught, far greater in its significance for humanity than either atomic energy or the control of the infectious diseases, has been the recent revelation of the magnitude and multiplicity of the disorders of human behavior and their fundamental responsibility for the unhappy state of the modern world. These overwhelming problems cannot be solved by a handful of psychiatrists. They have their origins in the homes and habits of the people, in their social and economic environment, and in their attitudes toward one another from birth to death. This sick world can be cured neither by psychiatrists nor by an army of practitioners of medicine. And so we physicians, in ever broadening appreciation of the importance of social medicine bring our burden to the people through public lectures such as these, and through individual instruction, in the hope that by better public understanding the means may be created for alleviating the spiritual as well as the physical ills of mankind.

The Academy is beholden to those who have contributed to this outstanding series of Lectures; to Major-General Norman T. Kirk, Surgeon-General, United States Army; to Dr. Arthur K. Solomon, of the Harvard Medical School; to Dr. René Spitz, of the New York Psychoanalytic Institute; to Dr. Nolan D. C. Lewis, Director of the New York State Psychiatric Institute and Hospital; to Dr. Howard W. Haggard of Yale University; and to Dr. René J. Dubos, of the

Rockefeller Institute for Medical Research. These are men who carry responsibilities which are the penalty of pre-eminent position, yet each has taken on the added burden of preparing and delivering the papers published in this volume.

To the Committee that organized these Lectures; to the Chairmen who presided at the meetings, and to our own Fellow, Dr. Orrin Sage Wightman, who contributed both in vision and in substance to the initiation and the advancement of these Laity Lectures go our particular thanks.

GEORGE BAEHR, M.D.
President, The New York
Academy of Medicine

New York
September, 1947

INTRODUCTION

ACH YEAR when the program for the ensuing series of these Lectures to the Laity is being planned by a Committee of the New York Academy of Medicine one of the questions which comes up for consideration is their niveau and scope. Should the topics be homely, practical, and simple, limited to certain phases of medical care and presented by well-qualified practicing physicians, or should the broader aspects of public health and medical problems be favored and covered by outstanding authorities not necessarily physicians. The latter idea nearly always wins out, not only because it is felt that there are available excellent popular books on the problems of the individual patient, such as regimes for chronic cardiac sufferers or diabetics, but because the Lectures are published and become a permanent record of the advances from year to year in far-flung fields of medical endeavor and investigation. The educational function of the Academy of Medicine is probably better fulfilled, therefore, if these printed lectures present the philosophic aspects of scientific advances of medicine to the leaders in lay groups such as ministers, teachers, lawyers, sociologists, social workers, and others whose interests touch closely upon medical investigation.

The lectures in the present, the twelfth series, retain the thoughtfulness, thoroughness, and scholarship of their predecessors. The content of this volume reveals a wide range of subjects—some of them only indirectly related to the role of medicine since the end of the second World War. It is questionable whether any really notable changes in the position or approach of medicine to individual or community problems occurred after the recent world war, or for that matter after any war. Even the task of the so-called psychological rehabilitation of returning soldiers followed, except in minor details, procedures well established in clinics which had been dealing in peacetime with the social and other maladjustment of persons in every walk of life.

Indeed, the Linsly R. Williams Memorial Lecture on "The Role of the Medical Man in the War," by Major-General Norman T. Kirk, tends to affim that remedies often popularly considered as wartime discoveries—sulpha drugs, penicillin, D.D.T., atabrine, immunization against many varieties of infection, as well as shock treatment and insulin relaxation for mentally disturbed soldiers and psychic catharsis under sodium amytal—were essentially only the application and testing with vast numbers of men procedures which had been more cautiously and deliberately applied among the civilian population before the outbreak of the war. Perhaps, too, the amazing efficiency of the Medical Corps of the United States Armed Forces, and the teamwork of the various medical groups during the hostilities and post-war reconditioning, so well described by General Kirk, may be considered to be only an extension of methods previously developed and tested in the better civilian hospitals of this country.

It is striking that one-half of the lectures are devoted to psychiatric investigations which had preceded the war but which were greatly accelerated and expanded by it. These psychiatric lectures, "American Pioneering in Psychiatry," by Dr. Haggard, "Are Parents Necessary?" by Dr. Spitz, and "What the War Experiences Have Taught Us in Psychiatry," by Dr. Lewis, deal with very different facets of the ever-widening range of psychiatric influence.

Dr. Haggard's historical address covers the inspiring

activities of Dorothea Dix, whose life work in the nineteenth century did so much to improve the mental hospitals and the care of the insane in the United States and to protect the legal rights of the mentally disturbed. It may be noted that the most effective part of Miss Dix's work took place during the peaceful decades preceding the Civil War and that it began in New England, a part of the country least affected by the war with Mexico or the spasmodic violent encounters which preceded the Civil War in border states.

In Dr. Spitz's lecture we have the benefit of the application of psychoanalytic thinking to a pictorial representation of the reactions of babies to the deprivation of love and attention. He reaches the conclusion that it is of the greatest advantage, psychologically and physically, for the child not to be separated from its mother during the first year of its life. However it is not imperative that "the mother" be the child's own mother. She may be substituted by "any person who treats the child as its own mother would." Dr. Spitz advocates the proper training in mothercraft of all young women as a means for the more efficient care of their offspring.

Dr. Lewis in "What the Wars' Experiences Have Taught Us in Psychiatry" points out that the experience of medical officers at all the induction centers for selectees and in the army reaffirmed how great is the number of young men in our population who are emotionally unfit for combat service and the strict discipline of army life.

For the first time, in this series we have a discussion of "The Atom in Medicine." This subject was presented by Arthur K. Solomon, Ph.D., of the Department of Physical Chemistry at Harvard University. Investigation of radioactivity which preceded atomic energy has occupied the attention of scientists for over half a century, and the new advances during the past five years with radioactive isotopes have given rise to the hope that we will be able to penetrate to regions beyond human sight for the treatment of a variety of diseases including destructive neoplasms. Our interest, however, is directed not only to the treatment but to the more important hope that these radioactive isotopes will make possible the tracing of basic chemical changes in the body which have hitherto eluded all analysis.

The final lecture is by René J. Dubos, a pioneer in searching for chemical agents derived from microorganisms useful in combating infections. His "Anti-infectious Agents of Natural Origin" deals with therapeutically helpful "natural products extracted from the biological materials and especially micro-organisms." This type of investigation, which has given us penicillin, gramicidin (discovered by Dubos), and streptomycin, is putting at the disposal of the practicing physician, even in isolated localities, anti-infectious agents inconceivable a few years ago.

These biotic agents along with atomic energy will all be used increasingly for the benefit of man in the post-war world, provided we can establish the indispensable sanity to employ the atom for our preservation rather than for destruction. Perhaps some help in securing a future of peace may come from the spread of psychiatric knowledge and the application of psychiatric methods and counsel to social problems. Eventually, psychiatric thinking may lessen human hate and aggression, and foster a more tolerant and kindlier relationship of man to man, nation to nation, race to race, and divert the impulse to destroy into the service of the moral equivalents of war concerning which William James so hopefully wrote.

C. P. OBERNDORF

New York,
August, 1947

CONTENTS

FOREWORD v
George Baehr, M.D.. *President, The New York Academy of Medicine*

INTRODUCTION ix
Clarence P. Oberndorf, M.D., *Chairman of the Laity Lectures Committee, Twelfth Series*

THE ROLE OF THE MEDICAL MAN IN WAR 3
THE LINSLY R. WILLIAMS MEMORIAL LECTURE
Major General Norman T. Kirk, *The Surgeon General, United States Army*

THE ATOM IN MEDICINE 18
Arthur K. Solomon, PH.D., *Assistant Professor, Department of Physical Chemistry, Harvard Medical School*

ARE PARENTS NECESSARY? 37
THE 97TH ANNIVERSARY DISCOURSE OF THE NEW YORK ACADEMY OF MEDICINE
René A. Spitz, M.D., *Member of the Faculty, New York Psychoanalytic Institute*

WHAT THE WARS' EXPERIENCES HAVE TAUGHT US IN PSYCHIATRY 54
Nolan D. C. Lewis, M.D., *Director, The New York State Psychiatric Institute and Hospital, New York*

AMERICAN PIONEERING IN PSYCHIATRY 69
Howard W. Haggard, M.D., *Director, Laboratory of Applied Physiology, Yale University*

ANTI-INFECTIOUS AGENTS OF NATURAL ORIGIN 92
THE GEORGE R. SIEDENBURG MEMORIAL LECTURE
René J. Dubos, Ph.D., *Member, The Rockefeller Institute for Medical Research, New York*

INDEX 107

MEDICINE IN THE POSTWAR WORLD

THE ROLE OF THE MEDICAL
MAN IN WAR

The Linsly R. Williams Memorial Lecture

⇥⇥ ✳ ⇤⇤

By Major General Norman T. Kirk
SURGEON GENERAL, U.S.A.

IT WOULD BE difficult to find anyone whose career
better exemplifies the role of the medical man in war
than does that of Linsly R. Williams. His record is an
inspiration to both military and civilian medicine.

Born in New York City in 1875, Linsly R. Williams was
graduated from Princeton in 1895 and received his M.A.
and M.D. degrees from Columbia University and College
of Physicians and Surgeons in 1899. He served on the House
Staffs of the Presbyterian and the Sloane Maternity Hospitals until 1902, after which he began private practice in
association with the late Dr. John S. Thacher. He was attending surgeon to the House of Rest for Consumptives
and to Seton and City hospitals, and also held several teaching assignments.

In 1908 Dr. Williams entered the field of public health,
and in 1914 he was appointed Deputy Commissioner of
Health for the State of New York. When the United States
entered the first World War, he resigned this position and
was almost immediately sent by the National Research
Council to investigate sanitary conditions in France and
England. He was commissioned a First Lieutenant in the

Medical Reserve Corps in June, 1917, and ordered to active duty.

He became assistant to the Division Surgeon and Sanitary Inspector of the 80th Division. He sailed with this Division to France in 1918 and served with it until October, when he was assigned to the Chief Surgeon's Office in the A.E.F. In December, 1918, he was assigned to the staff of the Commanding General of Civil Affairs in Occupied Germany, where his wide experience enabled him to develop quickly a broad program for safeguarding and maintaining the health of the area. A few months later he was ordered to Paris to assist the Red Cross and in April he was honorably discharged as a Lieutenant Colonel.

He succeeded Dr. Livingston Farrand as Director of the Rockefeller Commission for the Prevention of Tuberculosis in France. He carried the work already planned to a brilliant conclusion, and in 1922 he returned to the United States, beloved and admired by his French associates. He was decorated by the French and Danish governments. In October he was appointed Managing Director of the National Tuberculosis Association, in which capacity he served until December, 1928.

In January, 1924, he became Director of the New York Academy of Medicine, which high office he held until his untimely death ten years later. Those who knew him credit to his judgment and vision the selection of the present site of the Academy and the construction of its magnificent building; they feel that his leadership and personality contributed greatly to the Academy's high standing in American medicine today. An outstanding administrator, a noted specialist in preventive medicine, tuberculosis, and public health, Dr. Williams won the admiration and devotion of all who knew him.

His life typifies in a large sense the role of the wartime

doctor. Multiply his example thousands of times and you have a picture of the army doctor in action during the recent war. The life of Dr. Williams is particularly inspiring and interesting for its versatility. As Sanitary Inspector of his Division, he protected the health of the soldier; he played a big role in preventive medicine and, aside from his other civilian responsibilities, contributed to the research work so helpful to the army.

Not all of the 47,000 doctors who were in this war, at the peak, were Linsly Williamses. Fortunately, a large number were of his type, well trained, and specialists in their respective fields. American medicine's graduate training program, which has been in effect since the last war, gave us many more Linsly Williamses than would have otherwise been available for wartime service. This program has paid great dividends.

The high standards of medical care established by the Medical Department can be attributed to the many doctors from teaching staffs, who, like Dr. Williams, became the army's consultants. This teaching group in uniform were Medical Department consultants to the Surgeon General, to the Surgeon of each Service Command, Theater, and each Army overseas. They dictated the policies, arranged for the proper assignment of the younger specialist in the military-medical machine and directed the preventive health measures and the care of the sick and wounded throughout the gigantic Hospital System.

In order to raise an Army of some 8,000,000, it was necessary to examine physically more than 15,000,000 men who were called by Selective Service. The physically and mentally unfit, in the main, were rejected by this screening. Army medical officers were assisted in this great task by civilian physician volunteers. Many others found unfit for service while in training camps were hospitalized, restudied, reclassified, or separated from the service on Certificate of Disability Discharges.

It was at this early stage of induction that the Army for the first time began routine X-rays of the chest, a procedure that was largely responsible for the low tuberculosis rate. In the first World War the admission rate for tuberculosis was 12 cases per thousand per year; this was reduced in the second World War to 1.2.

From the time of induction until the day of discharge the Medical Department did everything possible to safeguard the health of the soldier. The battalion and squadron surgeons served as family physicians, vaccinated and innoculated him, gave instruction in first-aid and personal hygiene, made the routine monthly examinations, and then before shipment overseas gave him another complete physical check-up. To care for those who became sick, hospitals were established with sufficient beds in each training camp and overseas theater. During the war there were 15,000,000 admissions to Army hospitals.

Out of the 500,000 enlisted men and women in the Medical Department some 120,000 were trained as Medical, Surgical, Dental, Laboratory and X-ray Technicians and for other technical assignments. This training mission was just another assignment for the "Medical Man at War." Not one was louder in his praise of the medical-aid man than the doughboy who became a battle casualty, unless it was the present Chief of Staff, General Eisenhower, who said of him,

Unbounded appreciation and admiration were freely given by our fighting soldiers to their comrades who were armed only with stretchers and first-aid kits. These sentiments were best expressed by the unanimous insistence of our front line regiments that their Medical Detachments be awarded a battle badge equivalent in its implication to the one that decorated the combat infantry. A greater military accolade than this, no department, no service, no unit could receive.

The National Research Council, through its many committees of civilian specialists and through the Office of Scientific Research and Development, gave valuable advice and made many contributions to the Office of The Surgeon General as a result of research carried on in various medical schools and universities throughout the country. Thousands of new chemical compounds were developed and tested in an all-out effort to obtain a drug that would cure relapsing malaria. Results have been more than promising.

Penicillin had scarcely been tested as to its curative value. It soon became known as the wonder drug. Its value and limitations were proved by clinical and laboratory research. Prior to 1943 the world had produced a total of only one pound. Early in 1945 the original goal of 300 billion units a month, or 15 pounds per day, was passed. The original price of $20 per vial was cut to the present figure of approximately 76 cents for the same amount.

Streptomycin, another earth fungus, was a wartime discovery of Dr. Selman A. Waksman of Rutgers University, New Jersey Agricultural Experiment Station, New Brunswick, New Jersey. Its use and limitations in the cure of disease are now being studied by both Army and civilian physicians.

Our Army could well have lost the war in the Pacific to the mosquito as a vector of malaria. It was a formidable enemy in North Africa and in Italy as well. Early in the war, malaria was causing ten times as many casualties as the Japanese. Atabrine was found to be equally as good as quinine, which had been lost to us when the Japanese overran the Dutch East Indies. It suppresses all forms, and cures the malignant type of malaria. The death rate from malaria was .05 percent regardless of the early high incidence. With the development of repellents as the result of combined research, proper malaria discipline and control measures along with suppressive atabrine, the rate of infection was soon reduced to one fourth of the original incidence.

DDT, a chemical known to the Agriculture Department as an insecticide effective against the potato bug in Europe, was further studied as a shortage developed in pyretherum which was then being used for the control of insect vectors. Incorporated in a dusting powder it was soon proved lethal to the body louse, the vector of epidemic typhus; to the rat flea, the vector of plague; and, as the residual spray, to the fly—the vector of typhoid, the dysenteries, diarrhea infections, hepatitis and possibly poliomyelitis. It is also lethal to the adult mosquito and to its larva as well, whether sprayed over breeding areas from a plane or as a residual spray as in the case of the fly. Thus DDT assisted in the control of malaria, dengue, filariasis, and other tropical diseases.

More than a million people died of epidemic typhus in the Balkans following World War I. An epidemic threatened Naples just after its surrender to our Allied arms in the second World War. It was rife in German detention camps and has appeared in small epidemic proportions in Korea and Japan. Each outbreak has been completely controlled by DDT mass dusting.

American troops have been protected against the following diseases by compulsory vaccination or immunization: smallpox, typhoid, tetanus, typhus, cholera, yellow fever, influenza, Japanese B-encephalitis, plague, and diphtheria. All American troops are immunized routinely against the first three. Soldiers going to countries where they are subject to the others are immunized against them.

There have been two deaths from tetanus in immunized soldiers, none from yellow fever or epidemic typhus. The incidence of typhoid fever has been .03 per thousand per year compared with .37 in the first World War or about one twelfth of the last war's rate.

The Board for the Investigation and Control of Influenza and Other Epidemic Diseases in the army and the various commissions operating under it, composed of distinguished civilian consultants to the Secretary of War, was early established by the Preventive Medicine Division of the Surgeon General's Office. This group gave great assistance in the field of preventive medicine. It is now known as the Army Epidemiological Board. Its members isolated the virus, described the vector, and pointed out protective measures for the control of scrub typhus. This required extensive field studies in New Guinea. The Board also developed and proved through research studies an effective influenza vaccine. In a two-month period in the fall of 1945, on their recommendation, 8,000,000 men in the U.S. Army were given this protection by immunization.

The sanitary engineer controlled the incidence of waterborne diseases by purification measures involving filtration and chlorination of drinking water supplies. Added protective measures against recontamination necessitated an adequate residual of chlorine being carried to the point of consumption. Diatomite filters, an important development of the Corps of Engineers in collaboration with sanitary engineers of the Army Medical Department, are effective in completely removing amoeba cysts and snail parasites which cause schistosomiasis. Halazone tablets were used for the sterilization of water in the soldier's canteen.

Major Stanley F. Erpf, then Lieutenant, Dental Corps, developed the acrylic eye early in 1943 in the European Theater. This artificial eye, made of water-clear plastic and individually fitted and colored, has entirely replaced in the army the easily breakable, inferior, custom-made glass eye.

Liquid and dry plasma, which saved many American lives in this war, were developed under the auspices of the National Research Council. From this study of blood, blood derivatives and fractions, came gamma globulin, a protection against measles, and fibrin foam, used by the neurosurgeon in brain surgery to control capillary bleeding.

Plasma alone proved insufficient for resuscitation in the bled-out or badly shocked patient to permit life-saving surgery. It was necessary to supplement it with whole blood. Thanks to research, it was possible to fly whole "O" type blood from this country to the hospitals supporting the armies in the field, both in Europe and the Pacific.

A foreign-body locator was developed here in New York under the direction of Dr. Moorhead, which proved to be of great assistance to the military surgeon.

The neurosurgeon introduced tantalum in the form of fine wire for peripheral nerve suture, and plates were cut and fashioned from this inert metal to close skull defects.

This is the first war in which this nation lost more men killed in battle than died of disease. The over-all death rate was 0.6 per thousand men per year as compared to 16.5 in the first World War.

Thanks to penicillin and sulfa drugs, the mortality from pneumonia has been reduced from 24 percent to 0.6 percent. Likewise the death rate in meningitis has been reduced from 38 to 4 percent. Days lost from venereal disease have been reduced from 46 to 4, in an average case, and the complications have likewise declined. Unfortunately, the incidence of infection has increased, both in the civilian and military population since the war.

Newer methods in the treatment of the psychotic patient with electric shock and controlled insulin have greatly reduced the morbidity rate; many more patients return to their homes, with at least a social recovery. The barbituates, properly used, have assisted the psychiatrist in the treatment of the battle-fatigued and emotionally disturbed patient.

Of the 599,000 battle casualties that our army suffered, 377,000 were returned to duty in the theater; only 4 percent, or 27,000, died of wounds. Of those who were evacuated to the United States for definitive care, some 60,000 more were returned to duty; 10,000 still remain under treatment. Most of the others have been discharged from the service and have returned to their places in civil life.

Prompt surgery, aided by penicillin, the sulfa drugs, whole blood and plasma, together with new and improved surgical techniques, was responsible for saving the lives of 96 percent of the wounded who lived to reach a hospital. Surgery was taken to the man at the front. Medical-aid men accompanied combat troops into action, administering to the wounded where they fell. Field-hospital platoons supplemented by surgical teams operated on the non-transportable at the clearing station in the division area.

Surgical care was divided into three echelons: Initial or primary surgery was performed in forward hospitals. Wounds were thoroughly debrided, left open, immobilized by plaster or splints, and made ready for transportation to fixed hospitals in the rear. Resuscitation is necessary at this echelon of treatment. Most of these patients are in shock and many have lost much blood.

At the fixed hospital in the rear, intermediate or reparative surgery was carried on. Here, plaster and splints were removed, secondary closure was accomplished by plastic procedure or by skin graft, fractures of long bones were placed in suspension traction until consolidated, and then fixed in plaster for transportation to the United States. Soft tissue wounds healed much earlier under these procedures, and the soldier was returned to duty in the theater in a much shorter period of time. Compound fractures were converted into simple fractures and arrived home without osteomyelitis and with advanced union. Colostomies, which had been performed as a life-saving measure when initial surgery was done, were prepared for the patient's evacuation to the United States or closed in the theater. Thoracotomy for the removal of blood clot or foreign bodies became routine, and many of these patients returned to duty in the theater; formerly they would have returned home with a drainage tube in the chest, with chronic empyema, marked loss of weight, and requiring extended hospitalization.

In the United States, and at time in the theaters, definitive or reconstructive surgery was practiced. Here plastic procedures on skin, nerve, bone, vessels, were carried on to correct the defect, to mobilize joints and prepare the patient for return to the army or to civil life.

During the month of May, 1945, some 56,000 patients were returned to our shores by sea and air. They were admitted to our debarkation hospitals on the coasts, many of them coming to the port of New York. On arrival at the hospital, each patient's name, with a code showing his home and his diagnosis, was wired to the medical regulator in the Surgeon General's Office, and within twelve hours a wire went back to the debarkation hospital indicating the hospital in the United States to which the patient would be sent for definitive care.

There had been set up in the Zone of the Interior 65 general and 13 convalescent hospitals to take care of overseas evacuees. This was in addition to beds available in station and regional hospitals in the United States to give care to the soldier-in-training at home. In Europe alone, there were 230,000 beds at the time of the Battle of the Bulge, 190,000 of these being occupied by patients at that time. In all, some 200 general hospitals were operating in overseas theaters at the peak, and at one time the load of patients overseas and at home reached 500,000. In the hospital system in the Zone of the Interior in August, 1945, there were 320,000 patients.

There were too few men who like Linsly R. Williams were specialists—in medicine and surgery and their sub-specialties—properly to man the overseas hospitals and those at home. In the European Theater hospital centers of three or more general hospitals were set up, and in this manner patients with a particular type of injury or disease could be concentrated in a designated unit and specialists in that field assigned. Here at home it was necessary to set up specialized centers in our general hospitals and to staff them with specialists who could give the best care to the wounded and sick. Among others, there were 3 centers for the blind, 3 for the deaf, 7 for amputees, 19 for neurosurgery, 2 for tuberculosis, 2 for tropical diseases, 9 for plastic surgery, 5 for thoracic surgery, 9 for ophthalmologic surgery, 3 for trench foot, 29 for neuropsychiatry, and 19 for neurology. All of these hospitals were staffed to give general surgical and orthopedic care. More than 60 percent of the battle casualties had extremity wounds. On arrival at the debarkation hospital the overseas evacuee was sent to the specialized center nearest his home which could give him the best of care for his particular needs.

With all the beds available in our general hospital system, we still had 90,000 more evacuees than beds. So a plan was devised whereby patients who were not too ill were given sick furloughs to visit their families at home.

The 1,500 blind patients went to two specialized centers to complete their surgery and to be given instruction for the blind. After the surgery was completed they were transferred to the convalescent hospital at Avon, Connecticut, where psychological adjustment to their disability was made. They continued their training in Braille and other aids to the blind and were also trained in an occupation or prepared to enter a civilian school to learn a new vocation.

There were 15,000 amputees treated in the seven amputation centers, where many had their stumps revised, were fitted with prostheses, and were taught to use them. Today there remain some 1,200 of these men who lost a leg or an arm and who are still receiving care. The medical man at war had to learn about the surgery, the fitting, and the care of the amputee. Practically none had had similar experience in civil life.

Under the able direction of Dr. Sterling Bunnell, of San Francisco, centers were set up for the care of the crippled hand, of which there were some 20,000 cases. Under his guidance many young surgeons were trained in this specialty, in which there are too few trained men.

To the 19 neurosurgical centers we sent men with brain injury, cranial defects, peripheral nerve injuries, and paraplegics. As pointed out above, skull defects were repaired with tantalum plates, the peripheral nerves sutured, and in these centers a program for the definitive care of the 1,500 paraplegics was developed. Before the war this type of patient, unfortunately, received little attention and his life expectancy, due to ascending bladder infection, was limited to months rather than to years. Too often these patients presented many bedsores, were underweight and poorly nourished, with superpubic drainage, bladder infection, and stone formations in the genito-urinary tract. A team was developed for their rehabilitation: the dietitian, who daily prepared meals with known calorie and vitamin content; the nurse, who gave 24-hour nursing care to prevent the further development of bedsores and to hasten the healing of those already present; the neurosurgeon, who again explored the spinal-cord lesion, when indicated for the relief of pain or spasm; the urologist, who by tidal bladder irrigation and the use of streptomycin cleared up the bladder infection, removed the stones, and assisted the patient in developing an automatic bladder; the plastic surgeon, who closed the bedsores either by full-thickness skin graft or plastic procedures on the skin; the orthopedic surgeon, who prescribed braces so as to make the patient ambulatory; and the ward officer, who became the family physician, and by his personality and leadership sent the patient out ambulant, in a wheel chair, or walking, to carry on daily exercises either in bed or in walking classes after being fitted with braces.

In the three centers for the deaf, new procedures were developed. Hearing aids were fitted under scientific procedure, the patient was taught lip reading, and his emotional reaction to his handicap was lessened by the attending psychiatrist.

In all these centers were many compound fractures, non-union from loss of bone substance, as well as soft tissue defects which occurred at the time of the original injury. The too-few orthopedists, in conjunction with the plastic surgeon, have done a remarkable job in the reconstruction surgery necessary to rehabilitate this group of patients.

The plastic surgeon in the plastic centers is still working on facial injuries, restoring a nose, a whole lower jaw, or an ear lost in combat or as the result of severe burns, or of frostbite encountered in high-altitude flying.

To the tropical disease centers were admitted patients suffering from schistosomiasis, a tropical disease little known in this country. The microscopic parasite enters the skin of the soldier who bathes in water containing the snails infested with the *schistosomiasis japonicum*. Relapsing malaria was most troublesome but the recurring attacks were very quickly brought under control with atabrine.

American medicine can well be proud of the record achieved by its doctors who headed the team and who were ably assisted by the American nurse who gave unstintingly and without thought of self in carrying out her nursing duties. The medical soldier, both male and female, in this country and overseas, also made an important contribution as members of the team.

I cannot close without speaking with admiration of the job done by the dental officer who became a member of the plastic surgeons team, made some two million men physically fit for induction by the correction of dental defects, and gave oral and surgical care to this fine army of ours. And, likewise, the veterinary surgeon rendered excellent service in the inspection of tons of meat and dairy products which were shipped throughout the world to feed our army.

The third phase of the rehabilitation of the sick and injured American soldier—physical medicine or reconditioning—accomplished remarkable results both overseas and in this country. Physical therapy had already demonstrated its worth in medicine in the first World War.

During the Tunisian Campaign in 1943, I saw a physical rehabilitation battalion in the British Army in a tent camp on the sand dunes of North Africa. Under the guidance of trained medical officers and male physical-training sergeants, soldiers recovering from wounds were toughened and readied for return to duty. To a lesser degree this program was getting under way in our army in the Mediterranean Theater of Operations.

A need was realized for an intensive program that would help the patient both mentally and physically in his recovery from illness and wounds. In the fall of 1943, the Surgeon General's Office initiated the army's reconditioning program. Gymnasiums were constructed at each general hospital, which included curative gymnastics focused on improvement of the specific disability—a bad back, a stiff ankle, shoulder, or knee. Convalescent sections were organized at each general hospital and, later, when the patient load grew greater, convalescent hospitals were established in abandoned cantonments to house 50,000 patients. Swimming pools were built and athletic fields enlarged and improved. Psychiatric patients were removed from hospitals and placed in companies and battalions in convalescent hospitals under the guidance of a trained psychiatrist and clinical psychologists. For diversional and prevocational training for the handicapped, large shops were established: machine, wood-working, and automobile repair shops. To the thirteen convalescent hospitals were admitted 212,000 patients. The limitation and type of physical and mental reconditioning were prescribed by the attending physician and carried out under his guidance. Later, educational reconditioning was added, under Information and Education officers, particularly for the handicapped before return to civil life.

Similar programs were set up for conditioning troops for return to duty in overseas theaters. Two reconditioning centers were operating at maximum capacity in the European Theater in the spring of 1944. This program was greatly expanded and won the praise of all line commanders, as well as medical, who saw the work done.

The overseas reconditioning program played no little part in returning to duty in the theater 375,000 of the 598,000 battle wounded. This is just an example and only a small part of their accomplishments.

Without adequate pre-war planning and with total lack of trained personnel and facilities to accomplish its mission, physical medicine "grew up" in this manner during the war period. The results were epoch-making.

THE ATOM IN MEDICINE

By Arthur K. Solomon, Ph.D.

THE MEDICAL use of the atom probably dates back to those early days when the Arabs, attracted by the glitter of that liquid metal, mercury, came to learn its medicinal qualities. By the middle of the fifteenth century, mercury was certainly used in the treatment of venereal disease, and even now, synthesized into simple inorganic chemicals, it remains of great value to the physician, though recent discoveries have diminished, in some respects, its importance.

It may appear that the atom, in the ancient sense, is losing out in the competition with more sophisticated remedies; however, in the modern sense the atom has been transmuted into a new and wonderful tool for the study of the human body. I use the word "transmuted" advisedly, because it is transmutation exactly as the alchemists foretold that endows the atom with these new properties.

In 1934, not quite four decades following the discovery of radioactivity by Becquerel in France, Irene, daughter of Marie and Pierre Curie, together with her husband Frédéric Joliot, discovered artificial radioactivity and proved that ordinary elements, not naturally radioactive, could be endowed with properties similar to those of radium itself.

The first two of these decades, from 1896, the date of Becquerel's exciting and accidental discovery of radioactivity, to about the beginning of the first World War, were occupied in discovering and classifying the properties of natural radioactivity. Painstakingly and hesitatingly the first few basic facts emerged. Three separate and distinct types of radiation were found to exist. Sometimes the radioactive atoms disintegrated with the emission of alpha particles; sometimes they threw off beta particles; sometimes they emitted gamma rays. The exact identification and characterization of these rays required skill and facility in detective work hardly exceeded by Sherlock Holmes.

Although it was long assumed that the alpha particle was the massive doubly charged nucleus of the helium atom, this proof was not finally accepted by the scientific world until a detectable quantity of helium was isolated from radioactive material and shown to have properties identical with normal atmospheric helium. Today we describe the alpha particle by stating that it has a mass of almost four and a positive charge of two.

But the principal actor in the drama of natural, and for that matter artificial, radioactivity is the beta particle, whose mass is only one eight thousandth of that of the alpha particle, and whose single charge is of the opposite sign, negative. Once properly segregated, the beta particle proved to be none other than the common or garden variety electron.

The third and final character is the gamma ray, which is no particle at all (in the classical or pre-Einsteinian world) but merely radiation of very high energy. Thus unmasked, the gamma ray emerges as an X-ray of abnormally high energy.

Once the characters of the drama were finally identified as old friends—the alpha particle as a helium nucleus, the beta particle as an electron, and the gamma ray as an X-ray —the significance of their roles began to emerge. Natural radioactivity is found, with two exceptions, in elements as heavy as or heavier than tellurium and lead. Uranium, recently become so notorious a member of the naturally radio-active family was, at least before 1939, the heaviest-known naturally occurring element. Elements as heavy as these do not seem to be able to hold themselves together so well as their lighter brothers; they disintegrate spontaneously throwing off the alpha, beta, and gamma radiations I have described.

Although they disintegrate spontaneously, they do so at a measurable rate. Once the rates were determined, scientists found that the rate for each species was an invariable constant. One gram of radium, for example, throws off 37 billion alpha particles every second. Nothing that man can do by the use of temperature however hot, or pressure however great, can alter the rate of this disintegration. The international kilogram, made of a platinum—iridium alloy, and proudly kept in France, is far less exact, for subject to the whims of pressure and temperature the kilogram is an accurate kilogram at exactly 4° centigrade and 760 millimeters pressure, and under no other conditions. In 1903, Lord Rayleigh was so struck by the invariable accuracy of the radium half-life that he constructed a radium clock, which, depending on the natural disintegrations of radium as ordinary clocks do on an escapement, kept absolute time when Lord Rayleigh was alive, and if the clock survives, still does so today.

The rate of disintegration can be most easily described by what scientists call a half-life. Half of a gram of radium disintegrates in 1,690 years, half of the remainder in the next 1,690 years, and so in unalterable progression throughout time until it has all disappeared. In nature, these half-lives vary tremendously. Radium is neither the fleetest nor the most slothful. Thorium has a half-life of 13 billion years, and thorium C' has a half life of about one ten-billionth of a second. The length of the half-life is a measure of the stability of the radioactive nucleus; the longer the half-life, the more nearly stable the nucleus.

These natural radioactive elements are linked together in three great families. As the elements throw off their alpha and beta particles they change and transmute themselves into other elements, whose charge, and sometimes whose mass, is different from that of the parent. No Plantagenet, no Tudor, no Stuart ever descended more exactly from royal father than do the members of these three radioactive families descend in an unbroken line in the noble progression from uranium, actinium, and thorium to lead.

With these facts established, and in addition with the two outstanding discoveries of Lord Rutherford (the first in 1912 of the atomic nucleus, and the second in 1918 of artificial transmutation), interest in the field of physics shifted a little away from natural radioactivity. To be sure, the particles emitted from natural radioactive elements provided an elegant new tool for investigating the atom. For example, in both of his great discoveries, Rutherford used natural alpha particles as his primary tool. Furthermore, detailed, difficult work went on in the measurement of the energies of the particles, in the hope that there would emerge some clue to what lay hidden in the massive central core, the nucleus of the atom. But like so many scientific riddles, once the great basic simplificatory facts had emerged, it appeared that the most interesting work had been done and the main current of research shifted quietly to a somewhat divergent direction.

Then, nearly two decades later, came two additional discoveries which turned the stream back. In January of 1932, Sir James Chadwick, then not yet knighted, discovered the neutron. Two years later, the Joliot-Curies, who had themselves just missed discovering the neutron, demonstrated and proved the phenomenon of artificial radioactivity.

There is a certain sameness as one reads scientific literature just preceding an important discovery. It begins with a confusion in the interpretation of observed experimental data. Theories get more complex and cumbersome. Then follows the discovery, which once recognized, sets all the scientific facts in order; out of the welter and complexity of competing theory, there emerges a simple explanation. Having once emerged it seems obvious to all.

Chadwick's neutron was difficult to find because it was a new kind of particle, having no electrical charge, and most methods of physical detection of small particles depend on observations that arise from the charge of the particles. The Joliot-Curies were hot on its trail and would probably have found it within a matter of weeks had not Chadwick just beat them to it. The neutron's mass of almost one is just about equal to that of the hydrogen nucleus. Recent theory seems to indicate that it is a transient particle decaying with a half-life which has not yet been measured. It is still a tough nut for physicists to crack.

Then in January, 1934, Curie and Joliot discovered and reported to the French Academy that when alpha particles from polonium, a natural radioactive element in the radium family—named in honor of Madame Marie Curie's native Poland—fell on aluminum, they produced a radioactivity which remained when the alpha particle source was removed. This induced radioactivity was found to have a measurable half-life of two and a half minutes. The emitted particles were positive electrons, called positrons.

Once the discovery had been made, scientists everywhere found examples of artificial radioactivity. Fermi and his collaborators in Rome used the neutron with great success, and found that element after element became radioactive after bombardment by these uncharged particles. Ernest

Lawrence in California used his recently contrived cyclotron to bombard further elements with deuterons (nuclei of heavy hydrogen) and extended the results further. Ironically, the Berkeley group had for some time been bothered by a high background of apparent radioactivity which they had been unable to account for. Until the Joliot-Curie results were published, this phenomenon had been accepted as an inexplicable difficulty present in routine measurements. Today, we know that it is possible to make almost every one of the 92 or more elements in the periodic table radioactive.

With this as a background, let us examine how these facts, these basic discoveries of experimental physics, have reacted upon medicine. The role of X-ray in diagnosis is well known, and its use, as well as that of radium and radon in the therapy of malignant diseases is established by long practice. I do not believe that the mechanism of action of radiation on tissue has yet been explained in a detailed and accurate fashion. Yet it can be described in a way which accounts for its success in the treatment of malignancies. Malignancies are characterized by the rapid and uncontrolled growth of cells in one form or another. Radiation is known to kill cells. Growing cells are selectively more affected by radiation than mature cells. So it is simple enough to describe the effect.

The problem is purely one of selectivity. The poison of radiation may be administered in large amounts, provided always the damage to normal mature cells is kept small. The effect, whether X-ray, radium or radon, is the destruction of cells by radiation, and its limit, the limits of selectivity of the method. If one could find a radiative poison that would attack only the malignant cells, the selectivity would be multiplied and we would be in a much better way to control the malignancy. But we do not attack the primary cause; we are not able to make the cell normal, and hence must kill those cells that are growing abnormally fast.

Here is where artificial radioactivity may make its great contribution. Let us consider the element phosphorus, which can be made artificially radioactive with the convenient half-life of 14.3 days. Normal, non-radioactive phosphorus, when taken in the diet, is immediately diluted in the vast pool of phosphorus already in the body. One can determine the *average* fate of phosphorus by measurement of excretion, of the fraction found in bone and other tissues. But one cannot identify the *immediate* fate of the dietary phosphorus unless it can be labeled in an unmistakable fashion. Artificial radioactivity provides just such a label, and hence a means for determining the metabolic fate of any phosphorus taken into the body. That is, we can now follow the phosphorus through the reactions it undergoes inside the body.

Long before the discovery of artificial radioactivity, Hevesy in Sweden had used the natural radioactive elements in just such a way. The action of lead on the body has been closely followed by the use of radium E, a naturally radioactive form of lead. Unfortunately, elements such as tellurium, lead, and uranium are not very physiological; that is, they do not play an important part in the reactions that take place in the normal human body. Consequently, the research was limited and except for a small body of determined scientists, interest in the field vanished.

With the advent of radioactive phosphorus,[1] it revived

1 This information on phosphorus, as well as that on iodine therapy which follows, is taken from a report authored jointly by Dr. C. P. Rhoads, Director of the Memorial Hospital in New York, and myself, and issued in Part I of the "Scientific Information Transmitted to the United States Atomic Energy Commission by the United States Member," on June 14, 1946.

and flourished again. Using this new tool, it was easy to show that phosphorus given by mouth in the form of simple inorganic sodium phosphate was concentrated selectively in the bone marrow. Immediately, hopes rose that this might lead to a new treatment of leukemia, a fatal disease accompanied by a tremendous rise in white blood corpuscles. One particular kind of leukemia, related to the overformation of white blood cells in the bone marrow where many of them are made is called myelogenous leukemia; in common with all other types of leukemia, it is fatal. The treatment that obviously suggested itself was the use of radioactive phosphorus in order to localize the irradiation in the bone marrow and hence attack the malignant cells selectively. As if to make the prospect more alluring, these early studies also revealed that malignant cells took up radioactive phosphorus even more rapidly than did normal cells. Since the malignant cells are, in general, growing at a rapid rate, it is not surprising that they take up phosphorus more avidly than do normal mature cells.

Initially, the results of human treatment were encouraging, so encouraging that even those of us on the outskirts of the field were delighted to be taking a hand in these dramatic experiments. Almost everyone who has worked with a cyclotron can remember long hours of bombardment of phosphorus for use in emergency cases. We all felt well rewarded for our time because some of these early results seemed to indicate that life was prolonged beyond the ordinary course of the disease.

However, evaluation of results of new forms of treatment necessarily takes a long time, particularly in the case of chronic myelogenous leukemia, in which the average extension of the patient's life by X-ray treatment is six months. Unfortunately, the results do not bear out the earlier optimism. Life, to be sure, can be prolonged for a period; but for no longer than the six months' average after conventional X-ray treatment. Phosphorus therapy seems only to eliminate radiation sickness, that undesirable side effect so often associated with X-ray treatment.

Not only did the early experiments show that phosphorus was selectively absorbed in the bone marrow, they also proved that a similar concentration was exhibited in the lymph glands. The lymph glands are also active in the formation of white blood cells, and like the bone have an associated malignancy called lymphatic leukemia, also uniformly fatal, but somewhat more tragic, since this form of leukemia often attacks children.

In leukemic patients, the lymph glands take up phosphorus much faster than in healthy patients. Nonetheless, in this type of leukemia too, the initial optimism was not confirmed by eventual cure. The result of phosphorus therapy is no more encouraging than is that afforded by conventional treatment with X-rays.

In spite of the rather bleak position of phosphorus therapy in the treatment of leukemia, there is one disease which may be attacked, and that with remarkable success, by radioactive phosphorus: polycythemia vera, an overactivity of red blood corpuscle formation, not a direct, but a contributory cause of death. Since the red blood cells are also formed in the bone marrow, we might, using the same reasoning as we did for leukemia, expect radioactive phosphorus to control the rate of red blood cell formation. It is pleasant indeed to report that phosphorus therapy results in almost complete remission of polycythemia vera. To be specific, doses of the order of 10 millicuries of radioactive phosphorus per patient have resulted in disappearance of symptoms lasting up to two years without further treatment.

We now have experimental evidence that the red and

white blood cells are particularly sensitive to radiation, for many of the citizens of Hiroshima have died from aplastic anemia, that is their red and white blood cells have virtually disappeared. Dr. Aub, Director of the Medical Laboratories of the Huntington Memorial Hospital in Boston, has pointed out that Nature may have been aware of the extra sensitivity of the blood cell formation mechanism because it is so neatly packaged in the marrow of the bone where it is protected by a good hard case.

Iodine has also been used extensively with equally dramatic results in the treatment of disease. The well-known affinity of the thyroid for iodine suggested that radioactive iodine should prove valuable for the treatment of thyroid disorders. Perhaps the most striking case of the use of radioactive iodine was illustrated in a case at the Montefiore Hospital, in New York City. In the course of treatment for thyroid cancer, the patient's thyroid gland had been removed surgically. However, he still showed signs of overactivity of the thyroid, which were attributed to small local cancerous deposits of thyroid tissue, called metastases, distant from the original site of the thyroid but still capable of overexercising the thyroid's normal function. These deposits were shown to pick up iodine; in fact, they picked up enough radioactive iodine so that detection of the characteristic iodine radiation served to discover them. Thereupon, the patient was treated with radioactive iodine so successfully, I am informed, that now, some years later, he is still under good control.

Thyroid cancer, however, is a rare disease. Its incidence is only $\frac{1}{2}$ in every 100,000 in the population; a figure to be compared with the annual death toll due to cancer of 108 in every 100,000. Furthermore, only about 15 to 20 percent of the patients suffering from this disease are amenable to treatment with radioactive iodine. The facts have been expressed most succinctly in a speech of Dr. C. P. Rhoads to the United Nations Technical Sub-Committee on Atomic Energy:

It is a very interesting thing that as cancer cells become more and more unlike their parent cells, they simultaneously lose to a greater and greater degree the ability to share with the parent cells the function of selecting iodine and concentrating it in their bodies. In other words, the more malignant, the more vicious, the more widespread and destructive the cancer is, the less by and large, is its ability to pick iodine out of the blood stream and to concentrate it in the cellular structure.

Radioactive iodine, like phosphorus, has been most successful in the treatment of a non-cancerous disease—in this case, hyperthyroidism, a dangerous overactivity of the thyroid gland, often involving a considerable increase in the size of the gland itself.

Details of the exact dosage and the exact conditions of treatment of hyperthyroidism are still actively discussed. But, in the main, there is a wide body of agreement, amply supported by enough clinical evidence to justify the statement that radioactive iodine is highly effective as a cure for some 80 percent of the patients suffering from hyperthyroidism.

To summarize the results of what we may call radioactive therapy, two elements have proven to be therapeutically the most useful: phosphorus, and iodine. Each has served in the treatment of one form of cancerous disease, and one non-cancerous: phosphorus for the treatment of leukemia, with results no better than conventional X-ray treatment; and for the treatment of polycythemia vera with marked success. In the case of iodine, therapy of thyroid cancer is encouraging; treatment of hyperthyroidism is almost uniformly successful.

An attempt has been made to establish an absolute figure for the amounts of radioactive iodine and phosphorus required to make treatment available to every patient in the United States who might be expected to respond. A rough compilation of incidence rates, coupled with the percentage of patients amenable to treatment and the total dose per patient, yields an annual requirement of 380 curies of iodine and 330 curies of phosphorus. A curie is an amount of radiation equivalent to that given off by one gram of radium, which before the atomic bomb, sold commercially for $25,000 per gram.

The United States Government has been doing fine work through the Atomic Energy Commission in making large quantities of radioactive isotopes available to scientists qualified to use them in research and therapy. At present, the hundreds of curies of the annual requirement are greater even than the supply available from the government at its laboratories in Oak Ridge. Still, when the demand warrants this great supply it seems likely that such quantities can be made available.

So much for therapy up to the present. In this initial stage we have contented ourselves with the administration of radioactivity in simple inorganic combination: phosphorus as sodium biphosphate, and iodine as sodium iodide. The recent wartime advances in chemotherapy, coupled with an ever-increasing biological knowledge of the body, indicate that it is not impossible that we may discover chemical compounds which react preferentially in certain organs of the body. That is, there is a slim chance that we may obtain our selectivity by chemical means. Once having achieved this, it should be possible to attach the requisite dose of radioactivity to the selected molecule and introduce it to the body to make its own way, radar-like, to the selected victim. To further the analogy with radar, small amounts of radioactivity can be used as tracers to give us our initial information about the fate of our chosen chemicals. This effective combination—chemotherapy for selection and radioactivity for treatment—should now be actively explored, as an outside chance for a new approach.

The all-important factor of selectivity also regulates the treatment of cancer by X-rays. The problem is the same, to damage a selected portion of diseased tissue at the least possible cost to the adjacent normal tissue. Soon after the discovery of the neutron, and most particularly after it became apparent that neutrons could be manufactured by the cyclotron, attempts were made to investigate them as an alternate means of irradiation. As I have said, the exact method of action of X-rays on tissue, and this is true of alpha and beta rays too, is not yet clearly understood; it is agreed, however, that the effect depends on the density of ionization, roughly the resultant electrical energy liberated within the tissue.

The disadvantage of X-radiation arises from the fact that the X-ray ionizes more or less uniformly along its track, and that it is almost impossible to produce a dense region of ionization inside the body without subjecting the skin and all the intervening tissue to their due share of irradiation. There are, indeed, many effective schemes which tend to minimize the surface effect and increase the internal effect in the malignant tissues, but none which can eliminate the excess radiation completely.

The uncharged neutron does not itself ionize, but it can produce ionization by a secondary effect. When a fast-moving neutron hits one of the numerous hydrogen nuclei in the tissue, it tears the hydrogen loose from its moorings, and propels it rapidly through the surrounding tissue. The hydrogen nucleus, that is the proton, being charged can produce ionization, and thus in effect do the neutron's work. It was legitimate to expect that the neutron, which goes through matter with the greatest of ease, would be able to penetrate the skin easily Once inside, the neutron would produce, by collision, a most appreciable depth dose. Clever as the idea was, it didn't work. It appears at present, at any rate, that irradiation with fast neutrons does not produce an effect demonstrably superior to that of X-rays, at least in the treatment of cancer.

But there are other methods of tackling the same problem. For example, it is possible to accelerate protons directly; Ernest Lawrence, the Nobel Prize winner responsible for the invention of the cyclotron, is planning to extend the power of that legendary and marvelous machine to produce protons of some 200-million electron-volt energy. The completion of this cyclotron has been announced.

Nature has been very kind to us in the matter of the ionization produced by protons. At very high energies, let us say the 200-million electron volts which Ernest Lawrence expects his machine to produce, the ionization produced by the proton is very small, and it remains small until the proton has been slowed down almost to a stop. And then, at the end of its track, almost all the ionization appears at once. The neutron experience should make us cautious in predicting any marvelous advances, but the neutrons that we have had available never had nearly enough energy to propel protons to voltages approaching 200-million electron volts. It is fair to hope that when this new vast cyclotron gets to work, we will be presented with a small closely packed and sharply defined region in which we can obtain massive densities of ionization. Furthermore, we may reasonably expect to adjust the position of this small region of dense ionization virtually at will within the body. The new cyclotron is rapidly approaching completion. In a year's time we should know whether these possibilities are likely of realization.

In medicine there is one further field, one application of radioactivity in which the surface has hardly been touched.

I have mentioned one remarkable case of thyroid cancer in which secondary growths apart from the thyroid itself were first located and then treated with radioactive iodine. In a September, 1940, issue of *Science,* there was a stimulating report describing observations of the uptake of radioactive phosphorus as a diagnostic index. A remarkable correlation has been observed between the rate of uptake of phosphorus and the presence of malignancies. Since we know that cancerous cells grow much faster than normal cells, the results are not surprising, but it is nonetheless heartening to be able to detect cancer in this fashion, using its one unvarying feature—its rapid rate of growth—to make it give itself away, possibly well in advance of the appearance of any palpable growth.

The use of tracer elements marked by radioactivity makes it possible to accrue exact facts about metabolism that have not hitherto been accessible. By feeding or injecting a radioactively marked precursor we can, by determining the activity of one of its metabolic products, determine exactly the rate at which this product is formed in the normal body, and establish the limits in this rate which are observed in healthy individuals. So many internal disorders are metabolic disorders. The biological synthetic mechanism may be out of kilter in a number of ways, turning out its product too fast, too slow, or not at all. Since the body can adapt itself so wonderfully to cope with unexpected changes, the inspection system, in this case pain, may accept inferior products without active complaint. But once we have established proper controls, radioactive inspection may permit far surer and earlier diagnosis of metabolic ailments.

Having now summarized the diagnostic and the therapeutic aspects of the atom in medicine, I would like to turn to the subject of research, that aspect which is to me, at least, the most exciting of all the applications of the atom in extraneous fields. The application of the principles of basic research in the field of medicine is somewhat different from any other field. For in medicine, no doubt because the spectacle of human suffering is so distressing, there are two parallel paths to the relief of such suffering. One is the immediate, the pragmatic, the constant search for a cure of any kind. The second is the basic investigation of the fundamental metabolic processes. Since the first seems so often to produce immediate results, often dramatic, usually convincing, there are many who feel that it alone is the essential, and the second more labored approach is to be encouraged only if all other methods fail.

My point of view is exactly the contrary. I feel that on a broad front it is only possible to advance in medicine when this advance is grounded on a sure and steady increase in our knowledge of the basic reactions that take place inside the human body. To be sure there have been, and there will be, many observations based on our as yet incomplete knowledge which will provide means of curing specific ills. These are to be encouraged, these windfalls which become available to fortunate and determined investigators. But the windfalls will disappear, unless the active search for a cure is accompanied by advances in what we can call basic biochemical and physiological knowledge.

It is clear from what I have already said, that the atom in the form of its radioactive isotopes is an unparalleled tool for the investigation of basic biochemical and physiological processes. Work with the atom along these lines has been carried out all over the world—but I would not be far wrong in stating that the greatest advances arising from this new tool came from the laboratory of the late Rudolf Schoenheimer at Columbia University. Before radioactive elements were available, he worked with stable isotopes. A stable isotope—heavy hydrogen is the best-known example

—is an abnormal form of the element, usually heavier than the normal element as found in nature. Although the body is unable to distinguish between the normal and heavy forms, this difference can be detected by delicate physical means. Working with these isotopes, particularly heavy hydrogen and heavy nitrogen, Schoenheimer and his group undertook a brilliant series of experiments to investigate the behavior of the fat in the body.

They soon unearthed a fact which had hitherto remained unsuspected; namely that the fat is in a constant state of exchange. Continually the deposits of fat are being built up and torn down, new molecules are synthesized and old ones are broken up. However real and unchanging the pot-belly seems to its owner, the facts are that the fat within it is constantly in a state of flux. These results are summarized by Schoenheimer in a little book called *The Dynamic State of Body Constituents*.

I cannot here report in detail the difficulties which Shoenheimer had in discovering these new facts, but I can report in some detail the difficulties our group at Harvard found in investigating the method of formation of glycogen, that handy body storehouse of energy, a complex storage form of sugar manufactured in the liver. These experiments were undertaken in 1939 and 1940 and were based initially on a suggestion of President Conant of Harvard. He proposed a new method of glycogen synthesis which he believed might be correct. We are now all agreed that if we had been presented with a true knowledge of the difficulties at the start, we never would have been bold and innocent enough to have embarked on them. As it was, the experiments were a combined operation requiring the efforts of three biochemists, an organic chemist, and a physicist. Let me get ahead of my story enough to say that we discovered a lot of unexpected and fascinating facts, almost the first of which was that President Conant's initial hypothesis was wrong. In all fairness I must add that ours were too.

In those days we worked with carbon 11, a radioactive form of carbon that decays with a half-life of just over twenty minutes. The arithmetic that arises from its radioactive decay is most illustrative. Let us start out with an amount, x, of carbon 11. If we do not lose any of it chemically or in any other fashion, after one hour, we will have only $1/8\, x$, after two hours, $1/64\, x$, after four hours, $1/4000\, x$, after six hours $1/250,000\, x$. So largely we ran a race against time. Carbon 11 is made in a cyclotron by bombarding boron. We took the boron target to the chemical laboratory as fast as we could, separated the carbon from it, and then synthesized this carbon into lactic acid. Normal organic syntheses are carried out to obtain the highest yields, but we needed to obtain the fastest yields. If we could finish twenty minutes sooner, it was an acceptable equivalent for twice as good a yield. As a matter of fact, we were able to make our radioactive lactic acid in a period of from two to two and a half hours.

Thereupon, we fed the lactic acid to the rat—and to make sure he wasted none of our precious material, we fed him by stomach tube—an operation which even a fasted and presumably hungry rat does not relish. Then following a **period** of comparative calm, for we allowed the rat two hours and a half to convert the lactic acid he had so grudgingly swallowed into glycogen in his liver. This was followed by a period of feverish activity. The rat was sacrificed, and the glycogen extracted from his liver. The moment it was ready, we put it under the counter and all held our breaths to see if there were any detectable radioactivity in the glycogen. Our margins of time were so small that we could never be sure after a day's intensive work whether we would get an answer or not.

There were so many things that could and did go wrong. More often than anything else, the cyclotron did not work— or else it didn't work well enough to give us the necessary activity to start with. Moreover, rats, good pedigreed rats, are subject to peculiar diseases. We lost them from pneumonia; we lost them from heat prostration. At best, these rats are not tame; one of our number became very ill indeed from rat-bite fever. But we learned over those two years a great many new facts about gylcogen formation. The picture is very complicated, and the final details are still not completely known, so I will not attempt to present these experimental results now. But there was one fact, hitherto unknown, which we learned almost by the way, that rats incorporate carbon dioxide into glycogen. Carbon dioxide, that exhaled "waste product," is used as a building block in the formation of glycogen in the liver.

Today, fortunately, we can find out similar facts with much less trouble. For the Atomic Energy Commission's experimental pile at Oak Ridge, Tennessee, produces isotopic riches on a scale far greater than was possible with cyclotrons before the war. In particular, large quantities of carbon 14, another radioactive isotope of carbon with the delightful leisurely half-life of more than 5,000 years, are now available for purchase from the government.

In conclusion, my own feeling is that the most enchanting vista of the atom in medicine is in the field of pure research, a field in which we have been presented with a technique, that, like the microscope itself, will enable us to penetrate to regions hitherto beyond human sight.

ARE PARENTS NECESSARY?

The 97th Anniversary Discourse of the New York Academy of Medicine

⇥ ⇥ ✳ ⇤ ⇤

By René A. Spitz, M.D.

EXACTLY a century ago a committee was founded by a few of the most prominent physicians of New York for the purpose of creating a leadership capable of steering the profession of medicine through the troubled waters of the time. This Committee succeeded in organizing the Academy of Medicine, which in the course of the hundred years of service has gained world-wide recognition for itself and for American medicine.

The Academy was created as a result of new viewpoints in therapy which were fundamentally revolutionizing the medical approach to the patient. We are at the present moment witnessing another fundamental change in the medical approach to the patient, through the introduction of psychiatric thinking into every field of medical endeavor, be they as widely separated as internal medicine and orthopedics.

True to the tradition of its founder, The New York Academy of Medicine is in the vanguard of these new developments in medical science, both with the purpose of insuring the scientific reliability of the results offered and of disseminating that which is valuable in the new approach.

It is to this role of leadership that I am indebted for the

privilege of presenting some of the results of psychiatric investigation in a field not usually connected with psychiatry—that of pediatrics and child care. It is particularly the latter, child care, on which I would like to focus attention. For child care, and the forms it takes, are a function of society and of the social organization of the given moment.

Actually I cannot offhand conceive of any field in which the function of the given social attitude is expressed more forcibly and more effectively than in child care. By "effectively" I do not mean that the results are in concordance with the professed aims voiced. Results, after all, depend on the efficiency of the methods used; since these methods have to be applied to human beings, young and old, and since in the human race there is a strong element of contrariness, the results are often surprisingly at variance with the expectations.

However, the fact remains that nowhere in the whole society is such a large number of individuals exposed so helplessly to the whims of social trends ruling at the moment as in child care. Up to the end of its second year the human child cannot even voice intelligibly its disapproval of what we choose to do with it; it has to submit with more or less good grace. Unluckily, from the point of view of the general welfare of humanity, it submits with surprisingly good grace, thanks to the enormous adaptive capacity of the human race. Unluckily I say, because the consequences of this adaptability to measures which are mostly arbitrarily invented will show their consequences, often in a very paradoxical manner, months and years later; often, so much later that even careful studies have been unable to give definite proof of the suspected causal connection [we suspect] between improper child care and severe sickness in grownups.

In qualifying the measures of child care as mostly arbitrary, I refer to the fact that only a very few of these measures, outside the actual chemical composition of the food of children, are actually based on the welfare of the infant. They are instituted for all sorts of extraneous reasons: facilitating a normal social life for the mother by rigid adherence to a feeding schedule; making matters easier for the nursing personnel in the obstetrical hospitals by advising against nursing and for bottle-feeding infants; segregating newborn infants in a separate room without contact with their mothers, for the purpose of making the control of infections easier; and many others.

The strangeness of these measures will strike you immediately if you try to apply them to the grownup. How would it be for instance, if we were to segregate the City of New York in an aseptic enclosure for fear that persons arriving by train, by plane, by ships and by cars could infect us? We do the opposite: we do examine the new arrivals, but we leave the New Yorkers to do as they choose. How would it be, if because some people get indigestion after eating the usual food we all eat, it were decreed that everybody, from now on, must subsist on boiled milk and artificially produced yeast? Instead of this we inspect our foods. How would you like it if you could get your meals only at specified hours, on the minute, had a specified amount forced into you at that time and were forbidden to take a snack at odd hours when you feel hungry, just so that the restaurant personnel would be free to go for a walk or to look after other interests of theirs in the meantime? Without the possibility of substituting any other source of food and particularly drink? How *would* you like to stay thirsty, without a drop of water, from the time you are given your last drink at dinner until the time you get your first drink at breakfast?

All these things, which no grownup who had a say in the

matter would tolerate for an instant, have been inflicted on infants, along with many others that are much worse, though not quite as obvious. They have been inflicted and are being inflicted because it was possible to create a sort of propaganda that has penetrated all social strata unto the last home in the country. The powerful instrument of publicity on one hand, the widespread interest in medical, hygienic, educational information on the other, have created a demand for such information. This demand imposes on us responsibilities of a kind never before faced in the history of medicine and governmental care for public health.

It is the realization of this responsibility which has called into life in the course of the last 50 years an ever-growing body of investigation and research, the results of which are constantly being put before the public, applied, and then, if the occasion warrants it, accepted, modified, or rejected.

Such modifications are taking place, for instance, right now in regard to the rigid feeding schedule of infants; the self-demand method is being advocated instead. Modifications are taking place in the physician's attitude toward breast-feeding and toward leaving newborns with their mothers instead of separating them.

When it is a question of changing the attitude of the pediatrician or the obstetrician, the task is a comparatively easy one. However, other factors are at work, too, and their effect on the raising of infants is not easily controlled. I am referring to the factors implied in changes of a social and economic nature.

In the past hundred years or so our society has made a transition from the life of an agrarian nation to the life of an industrial nation. From decade to decade the momentum of the change has been one of increasing rapidity. This transformation has brought with it changes of a deep-reaching economic nature and has also modified the whole structure of the family. Theoretical efforts have been made to facilitate the adjustment to these changes. We are not concerned with these efforts; but we are concerned with one of the consequences of the industrialization of women.

An ever-increasing number of women have sought fulfillment of their lives less and less in the framework of the home and more and more in that of a job, a profession, or a career. The result is that the tasks of the woman in her home have been taken over by others, or have been organized in a manner to suit the requirements of the new situation. Appropriate theories of a social and medical nature have been created, in great part for the purpose of justifying the new development.

It is my belief that one of the factors operative in establishing the theory that the child should be fed according to the clock and not according to its needs has its origin in the desire to insure more freedom for the mother to take on a job. It fits well into the picture of a mother working in a factory, a child simply tucked away in a day nursery, where the mother will go to feed it at four-hour intervals. It fits very much less well into the physiological needs of the infants, as has been proved time and again both by pediatricians and psychologists in the last ten years.

The behaviorists' theory that the child should not be caressed, cuddled, or in any way petted by its mother also fits into the picture of the child deposited with the cloakroom attendant. Of course there were plenty of rationalizations. Foremost of these was that mothers were prone to "spoil" the child; that children who were indulged in the course of the first year were apt to turn into demanding, sniveling crybabies and into spoiled brats. Much of the thinking of the time was still influenced by the old adage of sparing the rod and spoiling the child.

Unquestionably the instances in which children were

being spoiled by their mothers had been on the rise at the beginning of the century. We suspect that this spoiling was simply a consequence of nature demanding her own. The mothers, having neglected their children for the whole day, were conscience-stricken when they returned to them and, under the urge of a strong guilt-feeling, overwhelmed them with caresses. It is only natural that under this regime of alternate deprivation and overindulgence the child lost its sense of direction and its feeling of security. That can only be ensured by a consistent sense of security in the environment.

The pediatrician who only saw the situation when over-indulgence was to the fore, strove to remedy the errors he saw. The result was that in the twenties we were confronted with mothers who did not dare to caress their children or to hold them on their laps. They relegated them to solitary confinement and only touched them for the ministrations necessary for purposes of feeding and hygiene. Small wonder that the medical world was confronted with a rising host of unfulfilled women who sought in arid jobs and restless social activities the satisfactions which were denied them in happy motherhood.

Small wonder that the children grew up into ever-increasing problems, with which the progress of education in the schools has been unable to cope. After all, none of you would be very happy if placed into solitary confinement for a year without any possibilities of social interchange or of a gratification of your emotional needs—but that is what we try to impose on our children! It is lucky that nature has provided sufficiently strong maternal urges in women to insure their disobeying the rules imposed upon them and permitting themselves to love their children, even against medical advice. In our country the trend of depriving children of mother love was luckily of short duration. A reversal of trends set in in the thirties and has become more and more accentuated in recent years.

Across the sea, in some countries, these theories of the parents' superfluousness in the infant's life have been pursued to their logical conclusion. Children in their first year were taken from the mothers, put into children's homes, and raised there without contact with their parents. The assumption was that parents are not only unnecessary to raise children, but that they are harmful. No information is available on the ultimate outcome of these experiments. The findings made in the course of our research tend to show that it cannot have been a satisfactory one.

On the problem of how to raise children in modern society, the United States has been outstanding, both in regard to the research done and in regard to measures taken by private groups and by government agencies to improve existing conditions. I need only mention the ever-increasing number of child guidance centers, of child guidance clinics, which nowadays are being established even in remote and rural communities; of the Child Guidance Bureau in Washington which distributes literature on the subject; of the research—psychiatric and pediatric—going on in our great hospitals; and of the numerous studies and publications by psychiatrists, pediatricians, and psychologists, both separately and in cooperative teams.

Today the consensus of opinion is that the child needs love and that the person to give it to him is his mother. It is not quite as widely known that the mother needs the contact with her child nearly as much as the child needs her. Neither is it quite generally realized that the father's cooperation with the mother is a necessary, I would even say indispensable, requirement for a healthy development of the child, as well as for the healthy development of the family. How this can be insured in our culture is a problem which I, in my capacity as psychiatrist, am not qualified to answer. I can only call attention to the laws governing infant development.

In the interest of ascertaining these laws I initiated in 1935 a research program on emotional development in infants. I soon realized that such research could only be conducted by a team in which both the viewpoints of psychiatry and those of experimental psychology were represented. I therefore included on the staff a child psychologist, Katherine M. Wolf, Ph.D., and at various periods technicians from the field of motion pictures, statistics, Rorschach tests, and so on. The investigations comprise short observations made on many thousands of children and long-term observations on a total of 275 children, for various periods, beginning at birth and exceeding one year. The populations investigated for such longer periods include: (1) children reared in their own families in this and other countries; (2) children reared under controlled environmental situation in various institutions in this and other countries. The method of investigation used for each of these children in the long term observations consisted in:

Developmental tests administered at monthly intervals and covering the sectors of perception, motor development, development of social relations, development of learning (memory and imitation), development of handling material (such as toys and everyday objects), and development of intelligence;

Observations at regular intervals of each child in its normal environment, totaling not less than 200 hours per year;

Construction of special experimental situations in which the behavior of the children was observed;

A case history containing: all data obtainable on the child and its parents prior to its coming under our observation;

the psychographs and developmental quotients obtained as a result of our monthly tests; the protocols of our observations; information on the child gathered in the course of regular interviews with parents and nursing personnel; when available, Rorschach of the mother; two photographs of the child taken at 6 months interval; the usual data as to weight, height, and so on;

Motion pictures of each child, recording its behavior in normal situations and any deviant behavior which might strike the observer at any time.

The data were correlated in the course of our research and processed statistically. These statistics on one hand, and the individual case histories on the other, form the basis of our conclusions and publications. I will summarize briefly the conclusions which we were able to reach. In these conclusions we speak always of the child's "mother." In so doing we do not necessarily refer to the child's actual mother. The term "mother" is applied to any person who treats the child as its own mother would, who gives the child the benefit of motherly feelings, of an emotional attitude and interchange which is innate in every woman and which is aroused in her at contact with a child, be she its own mother, a foster mother, or a nurse.

We have found that:

1. Children require during their first year the care of the mother.

2. If they are deprived of this care, disturbances of a psychic nature as well as sickness of a physical nature will develop.

3. The duration of the child's separation from its mother is of extraordinarily great importance.

4. The period in the first year at which the separation takes place is also of great significance. Specifically, it would appear, at least as far as we have been able to answer this

question with our present research, that the period during which the greatest damage is wrought by depriving the child of its mother (without providing an adequate substitute), is situated in the period from the sixth to approximately the fifteenth month. It is in this period that the duration of the separation becomes so important. It should be stressed that, when we speak of duration we are referring not to a few days but to weeks and months.

It should, of course, also be kept in mind that a statement like "separation from the mother has a dangerous effect on the child during a certain age period" is an oversimplification. It must be qualified as to the duration of the separation and as to the period when it takes place. During this early age the main source of stimulation is provided by the mother. A stimulus, to be effective, requires emotional reinforcement. If the stimulus lacks that, it does not become a stimulus at all. And emotionally reinforced stimuli can only be offered by persons who have some emotional interchange with the child—the mother, of course. Who else would trouble to give the child all the emotional stimulation it needs?

The consequences of separation after the sixth month take some time to show themselves. They usually are clearly visible after four weeks. By that time the child becomes depressed and weepy. After two months of separation it begins to reject the approaches of its environment and spends most of the time lying dejectedly on its face in its bed. Feeding disturbances appear, to which sleep disturbances are added, and a general decline in progress both as regards weight and as regards physical and mental performances becomes noticeable. After three months the whole process begins to take on the shape of a complete general retardation in every sector of the personality. The weepiness subsides, the child becomes more rigid in its expression, bizarre modes of behavior appear and the child becomes prone to sickness and infection. From here on, a progressive deterioration takes place, and, we suspect, becomes quickly incurable, resulting in children who remain all their lives severe psychiatric problems.

It is believed that separation from the mother after the second half of the second year is less destructive. It still causes serious disturbances, as has been shown by the work of Dr. Bender of Bellevue and Dr. Goldfarb, as well as that of Dr. Lowrey and that of Dr. Bakwin. But it appears that in the course of this later separation the chances of recovery are better than in those earlier separations I have described. The more the child advances in age and independence, the better it is able to tolerate the impact of separation.

For the purposes of the present study we will discuss two of the institutions investigated. In terms of the ultimate development of the children under their care, one of them succeeded in achieving good, the other bad, results. In the successful institution the children were cared for either by their mothers or by mother substitutes who looked after maximally two children. The babies of this institution, which in our publications [1] we have called "Nursery," developed into healthy, vigorous, active youngsters. Both mortality and morbidity were the lowest ever observed by us in any institution.[2] On the whole, the substitute mothers functioned well.

To this general rule there were some exceptions. They occurred in those cases where for unavoidable reasons the "mother" had to be substituted after the sixth month and the new substitute mother proved inadequate. The children tended by the inadequate substitute mothers showed in the

[1] "Hospitalism: An Inquiry into the Genesis of Psychiatric Conditions in Early Childhood, I," *The Psychoanalytic Study of the Child, a Yearbook,* Vol. I, 1945.
[2] "Hospitalism: a Follow-Up, II," *ibid.,* Vol. II, 1946.

course of the following three months a progressive impairment, the symptomatology of which we have already described.

In contrast to "Nursery," the successful institution, stands a second institution which we called "Foundlinghome." This institution, which is not situated in the United States, did not dispose of sufficient funds to provide an adequate number of substitute mothers for the children, though it does provide adequate food and every medical and hygienic protection that modern science has devised. In this foundling home the mothers nursed their children up to the end of the fourth month. After that the children came under the care of well-trained nurses. The only trouble was that the minimal number of children one nurse had to take care of was eight—this was only theoretical, because during the time I worked there, I saw no nurse taking care of less than ten or twelve children. Accordingly, these children enjoyed, at best, one tenth of a mother. This is tantamount to complete lack of social stimulation and social interchange; it represents a state of complete emotional starvation.

We followed 91 children in this Foundlinghome, two thirds of them from 3 to 18 months of age, one third, 18 months to 4 years old. The picture of psychiatric impairment we had observed in a few exceptions in Nursery progressed in the Foundlinghome children to truly tragic length. There were no exceptions here, or practically none. All the children were affected, all the children showed severe emotional disturbances. The longer the child had been under the motherless regime, the severer its symptoms.

On admission, the children in both Nursery and Foundlinghome showed a developmental quotient which corresponded to that of their age group in the cities of their birth. One year later the developmental quotient of the children in Nursery still corresponded to that which could be expected at their age. But the children in Foundlinghome were 30 percent below the average and by the time they were two years old their developmental quotient was 45. The progressive nature of the pathological process provoked by emotional starvation had reduced these children to low grade morons by the end of the second year.

The same pernicious consequences were manifested in the somatic sphere. Adequate nutrition was of no avail; the children in Foundlinghome showed quite inadequate gain in weight and seize. Notwithstanding excellent hygienic and precautionary measures, as well as assiduous medical supervision, they were susceptible to every kind of infectious disease. Finally, while during a four-year observation period not a single death was recorded in Nursery, in the course of two years in Foundlinghome the mortality was 37 percent.[3]

I am well aware that in these two institutions I have presented two extremes. It is obvious that the near total emotional starvation during infancy imposed on the children in Foundlinghome is hardly ever found in the baby reared in its own family. But it serves well to illustrate the importance of the mother's role at this early age. It is our concern that the socio-economical developments in our time tend increasingly to make it difficult, if not impossible, for mothers to fulfill this role.

You will ask what one can do to enable mothers in our modern culture to devote sufficient time to their babies. This question involves problems far too vast for an easy answer. I can offer a few of my own ideas, from the viewpoint of my profession. A comprehensive treatment of the problem must be reserved for more competent persons. But if I may presume by offering a few suggestions, I would propose that we organize the training of our future mothers. I

---

[3] "Hospitalism, a Follow-Up, II," *ibid.*

consider simply ludicrous our insistence on teaching future mothers every subject under the sun in preference to the most elementary and at the same time most urgent problems of their daily life; the answers to these problems are to be found in the subject—the science—the art of mothercraft, and this is taught in very few schools indeed. Do not misunderstand me. I am no advocate of the reactionary slogan "Woman's place is in the home." On the contrary, I think that woman's place is everywhere where she chooses to work and to function. But on the other hand I feel that there is one primary function of woman with which she should be made thoroughly familiar—and that is motherhood.

We speak glibly of the holiness of the family and we bemoan the passing of those close bonds which used to unite it. We complain bitterly about the falling apart of the family, which is supposed to be the fundament of the state. But what do we do about this, except to emit self-righteous exhortations addressed to the nation at large or to the children in our schools? It is not enough to proclaim from the pulpit the sanctity of the ties between parents and children, and that, as for sin, we are "agin it!" The close family ties, the loss of which we deplore, are a thing of our agricultural past. It is not from her own choice that a woman with a job is forced to neglect her children or to dump them in a day nursery, a procedure we consider undesirable before the beginning of the child's third year and dangerous before the end of the first.

But what is this mother of today to do? It is evident that in accordance with the changing social order the problem must be tackled in two directions. On one hand, appropriate economical security must be provided for mothers of infants to enable them to devote enough time to their offsprings. This is a project of such magnitude that I do not feel competent to discuss it. It has been discussed in many countries; measures—though not adequate ones—have been taken here and there to implement it, and it belongs in the field of social organization.

The second direction in which we could attack this problem is to provide in our schools a required course in mothercraft, to replace the knowledge which the growing girl acquired as matter of course in the agricultural family, but of which she does not get even the rudiments in our industrial civilization. Eighty and even fifty years ago, young girls helped their mothers and grandmothers in looking after the family and learned in this very practical manner their future job as mothers. Today, mother has a job and in most cases is not available for the purpose of teaching her daughter. Anyhow thanks to obligatory universal education the young girl has little opportunity to learn these experiences, since she is absent from the home too.

Why do our schools not step into this vacuum? And I do not mean that the schools should give only theoretical instruction in mothercraft. I mean that all young girls should have practical instruction in feeding babies, looking after them, handling them. I advocate a mothercraft internship for every young girl before she graduates from school. This internship should take the form of practical work in nurseries, orphanages, children's homes, hospitals and kindergartens. I first expressed this idea about two years ago. It is gratifying to me that similar ideas have occurred to a number of workers in this field and others, both in this country and in Great Britain. Dr. Strecker has just published a book on similar subjects and Professor Langmuir of Vassar has mentioned quite independently the idea of instituting for this purpose something in the nature of the "blood bank," namely a "time bank." Finally, the latest number of the *Journal of the American Medical Association* brings a report on an article by Dr. Young, Professor of Obstetrics at Post-Graduate School in London, demanding the creation of a new profession, the profession of a "Diplomate in Child Care."

Thus the subject is very much in the air at present. Isolated schools and colleges, one or two youth organizations, have in their programs attempts in this direction. But isolated attempts are not an answer to a nationwide problem. The existence, nay, the urgency of the problem, has found visible and tangible expression in the emergence of a completely new profession, so universal in our country that it has already become the subject of cartoons and comic strips, namely the "baby sitter." But this is no answer either. For the baby sitter is at best conscientious, but nearly always ignorant of the needs of the child. Other undesirable aspects to this solution are obvious and need not be discussed here. It is evident that besides moderate financial benefit the baby sitter does not derive the advantage in knowledge and experience which could be achieved if the whole problem were to be approached on a national scale, by our schools, and on the lines of some such plan as I have suggested.

It would be out of place to discuss here details of the time which should be devoted to such a plan, of the form the internship should take, and so on. But we can affirm that it would serve a number of purposes: it would facilitate the avoidance of damage done to children through lack of mother care in poor institutions; it would prepare our young womanhood for the most important task of their life.

At present only all too frequently our young women find themselves in the midst of their task as wives and mothers completely innocent of any practical knowledge, rushing to neighbors, friends, and family for advice, which then is given in a haphazard, helterskelter, confusing, and mostly very inefficient manner.

Proper training in mothercraft would give the future mother that security and authority which belongs to her as the pivot of the family. It would also give her the incentive to enjoy the children and the married life, and the capacity to do so. It might go a long way toward reinforcing in a practical manner the slackening bonds of the family. It might bring a solution to the problem of providing substitutes for mothers who have jobs which do not permit them to spend sufficient time with their children.

It may be objected that such a plan requires a vast organization and a great expenditure of funds. I believe such assumptions to be fallacious. The solution of these problems constitutes a large part of our obligation to our children, to the future generation, to the nation as a whole. It may also be objected that such a project will impose an unbearable sacrifice in time on adolescent womanhood. To that I will answer that the stake involved is human lives, the lives of the next generation. We do not hesitate to impose on the budding physician the sacrifice of at least one year's internship before entrusting the lives of our fellow citizens to his hands. I do not feel that the sacrifice we ask from our adolescent girls is any greater or that it is any less necessary.

WHAT THE WARS' EXPERIENCES HAVE TAUGHT US IN PSYCHIATRY

By Nolan D. C. Lewis, M.D.

WAR AND medicine have always been closely associated. The medical man tries, with every means at his disposal, to save the lives that others have tried to destroy and maim. Throughout history surgery has flourished and learned much on the battlefield, and other branches of medicine have been applied behind the lines in the struggle against pestilence and other forms of infections and diseases. In recent wars psychiatry has found its duties here also.

Man is well on the way to conquer every enemy but himself. With himself he has not made much headway because he does not understand his own emotional organization, and thus falls into his own traps. Psychiatry is the branch of medical science which deals with the mental welfare of human beings, or, to put it another way, psychiatry is the study of human adaptation. Like other medical specialties it has developed its own methods of approach to the problems of observation, experimentation, interpretation, diagnosis, treatment, and prevention.

Mental disorder and war are both limited to the human race, the former caused by some form of individual or personal pathology, and the other to social pathology. We do not need to be reminded that the proper study of mankind is man, and that total war sets a large number of new problems in adaptation.

In the first World War the medical officers as a rule were poorly prepared to cope with the emotional problems of soldiers. Many physicians not trained in psychiatry and others gone stale in army routine tended to explain emotional problems in terms of everything else under the sun, rather than in those of psychological conflicts. Their treatment and management of many of these hysterical conditions found its final solution in nothing but a pension for life.

When a war is under way, the psychiatrist finds many human problems in which not only are his services desirable, but, if they are not available, additional suffering is the inevitable result. In the military procedure, as such, the psychiatrist should assist in the selection of the recruits, should recognize, diagnose, and treat the early disorders appearing in the training centers and in the combat zones, should work on the problems of morale among the troops, and assist other agencies in the post-war period in their attempts to aid veterans seeking advice regarding personal matters. As far as the civilian population is concerned, mental health must be protected and maintained both for purposes of production and home-front morale. A host of children's problems incident to war need attention. Taken all in all, the job is too large to be accomplished by trained psychiatric specialists available to deal with it.

In wartime, community and public interests are placed before those of the individual. But we have learned that people break down under stress. Often, military service itself seemed to exert just enough stress to break the individual into a neurosis, thereby giving rise to the impression that some disorders are more common in war than in peacetime.

As war is the principal mental disorder of the civilized

world, and as the soldier must become a specialist in acts of violence regardless of how peaceful his previous life has been, the experience effecting this radical transformation ruins some, impairs others, and has little or no effect on still others. War is especially tough on those who possess a nervous predisposition. They may have to suffer great hardships when in poor condition to assume the burden. It seems that fear, fatigue, and injuries precipitate serious mental disorders principally in those who are predisposed in some way. Certainly, fear and fatigue joined together make a devastating combination for anyone to live with, in complete mental balance, and they are frequently followed by a period of depression.

The emotional cost of war cannot be assessed. The sorrow, grief, maiming, death, displacements, broken lives and homes, cannot be placed into statistical formulations. But occasionally some good things spring from evil ones. I refer here to the procedures in diagnosis and therapy that war has brought into the foreground for future use to the benefit of the people. Very little, if anything, has been discovered that is essentially new or revolutionary, but many experiences have modified our attitude and will direct our future. The proof and refinements of what we already knew and had in operation to a limited degree before the war have been made possible to the extent that we feel more secure in following them, and in insisting on the necessary reforms.

Twelve of every hundred men rejected at induction centers were involved in some personality problem; moreover, 40 percent of all medical military discharges were because of personality disorders (a total of nearly 400,000, but not more than 7 percent of psychotics admitted to the hospital were severely mentally ill), and another 150,000 because they could not fit into the army scheme. From all these rejections and discharges for mental reasons it became clear that a healthy physical body alone does not make an efficient soldier.

The experiences of the war reinforced our knowledge that some persons are constitutionally poorly organized to meet the ordinary demands of life, much less the pressure of military training and campaign life, although too many regular army men thought that passing a physical examination was about all that was necessary. To emphasize the point one need say no more than to mention the fact that better than half of all psychological troubles occurred in men who had never been in active service. The successful medical officer discovered that the patient was a person and not just a soldier who had developed a complaint.

We learned that although we had more trained psychiatrists than in the first World War, and a larger number of therapeutic procedures to try out, practically everything else was a repetition of the earlier experience and, moreover, that most of the neuroses of war follow the same patterns as those of peace. Some interesting reactions have been pointed out as being rather prominent and common in the second World War, such as urinary incontinence, goitre developing from severe emotional shock, asthma and hay fever tending to become aggravated, gastrointestinal complaints, and giant hives (urticaria). Sexual impotence was more common than among the civilian population. Of course tank warfare, anxiety, and pilot fatigue are new reactions not prominent in any previous war.

A crop of diagnostic terms or labels—"operational fatigue," "flying stress," "combat fatigue"—were sometimes given to psychoneurotic reactions to spare the men the disgrace of being called neurotics. There is considerable doubt that these acute reactions were actually psychoneuroses. It seems to me that many of them were merely the result of severe dilemma, instead of the more deeply seated and differently organized mental patterns of the psychoneurosis. These "dilemma" reactions have appeared in different forms in war situations from ancient times to the present day. Controversies over diagnostic labels and names are of little importance, as what we want to know concerns the facts of the *personality,* the *situation,* and the *reaction* so that we may take the proper measures to prevent and cure.

The failure in our educational system in psychiatry became very evident when the medical officers failed to recognize serious mental disorders, or placed them on some elusive physical basis that required prolonged hospitalization, loss of time, and unnecessary procedures; while in the meantime the disorders became fixed, chronic, and progressively more difficult to treat.

Severe stress over long periods may produce anxiety, conversions and depressions in an otherwise stable man. It is generally conceded that everyone has his "breaking point," that we all have one somewhere along the line, so that any one of us may be relatively weak or strong in this respect, without any reference to character, will power, morals, or to any societal defect. It is, rather, a matter of our constitutional organization with respect to all sorts of strains and responsibilities. This individual threshold or breaking point does not seem to be a fixed affair. In fact, it is conceivable that there may be persons who have none, in this sense, short of death itself. Is it the breaking point when the individual first starts to fail a little? Or when he becomes totally incapacitated and collapses? This point of failure in any given person is probably variable, changing from day to day and perhaps from moment to moment. It is dependent upon a great many factors of health, morale, and various other circumstances.

On the constructive side, war experiences taught us that even severe psychoneurotic reactions, when they are new and acute, can be treated successfully, if done promptly, and if there are no serious predispositions to emotional illness. If these acute cases are more deeply seated conditions, the removal of symptoms does not mean complete recovery. In fact, recovery is doubtful in the majority of instances. The fact that 60 percent of cases return to duty is no indication that the final prognosis is favorable. On the other hand, it was found that many personalities thought to be unstable functioned surprisingly well in combat and under other stresses. Also some neurotics gave a good account of themselves in battle but were unable to stand the chronic strain of campaign activities, with the regimentation, the discipline, and the dictatorial nature of the situation.

Between 1941 and 1946 there were about 1,000,000 admissions to neuropsychiatric services in army hospitals as contrasted with 97,578 in the first World War. Only 7 percent of these were psychoses, while 75 to 80 percent were neuroses or personality disorders. Among all of these the high (at least partial) recovery rate in the services was remarkable, as by 1945 seven out of ten went home rather than to a Veterans Hospital.

Among civilians in actually war ravished countries there were fewer mental disorders than might have been expected. However, there were increases in senile depressions and other senile psychoses following air raids on civilians. Curiously enough epileptics were not affected. Increases in seizures were not observed. There was a great increase in juvenile delinquency because of broken homes and disrupted families. In some countries this increased as much as 50 percent over peacetime. This particular experience may teach us that much of the security of the future rests on a good, solid, well-knit family life.

I shall now state briefly and specifically what lessons we have learned that should direct our efforts toward improvement in the understanding and care of mental disorders. None of these items is entirely new. As far as I can determine the war experience revealed no new principle. However it did produce elaborations, refinements, modifications, and contributions that consolidated much that was in the making and needing the test of practical application on a large scale, made possible only by a huge military aggregation of people.

I. I have already emphasized the roles of personality and predisposition to neuroses. We ask the question, is there a type of personality predisposed to war neuroses? What do we look for to detect predispositions?

In a study made at Walter Reed General Hospital and reported in 1943 by Colonel William C. Porter,[1] the past history of patients diagnosed as suffering from serious emotional disturbances revealed certain characteristics. Fifteen important ones were listed as follows:

1. Bed wetting beyond four years of age.
2. Thumb sucking or nail biting beyond six years of age.
3. Failure to engage in competitive games involving risk of injury.
4. Tantrums in childhood.
5. Abnormal shyness or sensitiveness.
6. Preference of playing alone.
7. Repeated grades, difficulty with teachers, chronic truancy in school record.
8. Abnormal fears.
9. Shunning of girls after puberty.
10. Faints.
11. Excessive autonomic system reactions to emotion; tremor, abnormal sweating, tachycardia, etc.
12. Sulkiness under discipline.
13. Abnormal attachment to mother after puberty.
14. Stammering.
15. Obsessional traits.

[1] "What Has Psychiatry Learned during the Present War?" *American Journal of Psychiatry*, XCIX (1943), 850. Reprinted by permission of the publishers.

A tentative evaluation indicated that the presence of six or more of these traits in the personal history should allow one to expect a breakdown under stress and that any four of them predisposes the individual to some degree of instability.

It would be interesting and perhaps informative to study this same group of characteristics in civilian psychoneurotics, checked carefully with similar studies on control groups including one group composed of highly successful persons who have been subjected to an equal amount of external stress. If further experience with civilian cases verifies these findings (and there seems to be no reason why it should not, as the material deals largely with the behavior of the early years of the patient), then we have important indicators at hand with which to work.

II. There is ample evidence to show that war problems have helped to perfect a number of brief psychologic tests that aid in rapid diagnosis. Many of these may be more widely used in civilian life, for example, in large clinics and in industrial offices.

Ten million men took the Army General Classification Test (A.G.C.T.). This was the most extensively used of the tests of ability, aptitudes, trade proficiency, and technical knowledge that were developed for aiding the army in classifying the personnel. It was an attempt to determine the ability to take certain types of training, and the capability of mastering kinds of tasks.

When these data are brought into relationship with the educational and occupational status, they will bring into the foreground our great national endowment of human resources, much of which is going to waste. It threw light on military problems as well. The test measures how intelligent the individual is, what he can learn, and the rate of speed at which he learns. *It tells what can be done now,* rather than what could have been done under better environmental, educational, and other circumstances—that is, it does not disclose innate ability.

It disclosed that there are large numbers of men whose levels of accomplishment in both education and job have fallen short of their real abilities and potentialities, and that we have in this country a vast amount of talent that is being only partly utilized, and this in a haphazard way. It is all very well for the economists and others to emphasize the necessity of conserving our fertile soil, our mineral, oil and forest resources, and with this we can only agree, but voices seem to be very feeble in insisting that we conserve this most important element of value, the intellectual capacities of our people. As it is possible now to select the most promising young people for higher education, for technical training, and for whatever form of future job adjustment that will yield the maximum for them, why not afford more scholarships, guidance and direction toward these ends?

Experience of the military services during mobilization and war dictates an expansion of civilian facilities for interviewing, testing, record keeping and counselling of young men and women. Staffs of qualified specialists such as those a few universities now maintain should be available in every educational institution to identify the most promising students and to facilitate their advancement. Incentives must be widely and plentifully supplied and new ambitions stirred.[2]

III. The studies on disorganization of behavior in fatigue states, in hysterical blindness, deafness and backache, the utilization of the mentally defective, and various other applications of military mental hygiene can be utilized in American industry, where many problems concerning employees are always presenting themselves for solution.

IV. Experience with the Rorschach test in the differential

[2] W. V. Bingham, "Inequalities in Adult Capacities: from Military Data," *Science*, CIV (1946), 152. Reproduced by permission of the publishers.

diagnosis of brain concussions and psychoneurotic reactions indicates a wide field of application and additional research.

V. The widespread opportunities to apply the electro-encephalographic technique to a variety of nervous and mental illnesses revealed a wider use and value in diagnosis and particularly in prognosis.

VI. There were at least four outstanding contributions to therapy, a field in which a great deal of experience has been amassed.

1. Psychotherapy under sedation proved itself to be a very valuable short-cut method—an abbreviated form of mental treatment. Sodium pentothal has been used freely in this work, but other drugs have also been effective.

Drugs facilitate the recovery of repressed and dissociated thoughts and experiences by rendering the personality less sensitive to the exposure of painful material which in the waking state may be very difficult to recall or almost impossible to face. In the state of drug sedation, interpretations and psychological synthesis may be accepted without any great disturbance. Resistances are thus circumvented. The more dynamically oriented the therapist, the better the results, as psychotherapeutic judgment is necessary here as elsewhere in mental therapy.

This procedure is called "narcosynthesis," and was used in treating certain war neuroses immediately after the breakdown. It brings relief from depression and anxiety when applied in civilian practice, and has been found helpful even in some rather long-standing cases.

Various drugs, including insulin treatment, and electric shock as well, without psychotherapy, are not likely to sustain a remission. Some form of psychotherapy is essential.

2. The use of hypnosis, which was applied also in the first World War, was revived and employed more extensively,

both alone and in combination with other methods. In the hands of experts it is a valuable type of therapy for properly selected cases.

3. Under the pressure of the necessity to afford as much help as possible to large numbers of emotionally ill people there was a notable improvement in group psychotherapeutic procedures, the so-called "Group Psychotherapy." Often treatment in the military services had to be done this way if at all. Group problems were thus handled and attitudes were changed. Treating patients in groups saves a lot of time and work but will the cures and improvements stand the test of time? How do they hold up? The same question may be asked of the widely applied shock therapies, and the answers must come with time and with additional experience and research.

4. There was an interesting and informative development of organized programs of living for neurotics during their treatment period. These programs utilized the techniques of individual psychotherapy, group therapy, and well planned educational, occupational, and recreational opportunities which were sufficiently successful to invite a similar trial in civilian hospitals. Psychologists, social workers and occupational therapists contributed extensively to this type of reconstruction.

VII. The military experiences reemphasize a long-desired improvement in administrative methods and facilities. They proved that efficient administrators of psychiatric hospitals and units must have clinical training in the specialty. They also proved that the urgent use of more auxiliary personnel is indicated, such as psychologists, social workers, occupational, recreational and educational therapists, nurses and attendants, who in collaboration with the psychiatrists compose the ideal working teams. Idleness on the wards led to relapses. Therefore the institution of this auxiliary personnel was deemed essential.

Adequate secretarial help to handle the necessary paper work incident to examinations, treatment, and research seems to be lacking in practically every hospital over the country, where anything active is going on.

From an administrative standpoint a revision of psychiatric classification, seemed advisable. A revamping of psychiatric or of any other established terminology is a large and complicated task. The result accomplished by the army in connection with giving names to acute combat conditions, personality disorders, and situational reactions for which there were no previous labels, can be used to some extent in the civilian practice of psychiatry.

VIII. War experiences, and the studies initiated by war, have reemphasized the desirability. of treating people before they are sick enough to go to a hospital. For example, there is considerable evidence that if schizophrenic breakdowns are caught early, as can be in military service, and not allowed to go along for periods of time, as they do in civilian life where eccentric behavior is more easily condoned, cures are easier and much more rapid. We as civilians should insist (not merely request) on the establishment of more child guidance centers and treatment clinics in the cities and towns over the country, that corrective measures may be available to those who seek for aid.

IX. Follow-up clinics for veterans and the establishment of small regional hospitals are among the most important of our urgent future projects. Perhaps the day of the large veteran and state hospital should pass in favor of more numerous tax-supported institutions, that will be smaller, more convenient, and more readily available to the populace.

X. We have learned from the war that a greater variety of patients with serious mental disorders could be treated successfully in general hospitals, especially when the disorder is in the reversible stages. In fact, the percentage of good results would have been high, if the statistics had not included the more resistant post-traumatic cases.

Floors or whole wings of general hospitals should be arranged to provide more facilities for cases of psychiatric disorder, particularly those in early and still modifiable stages. Here, in full cooperation with the internist and other medical specialists, it would also be possible to study carefully the psychogenic or emotional aspects of all types of convalescence, as well as the whole field of psychosomatic medicine, in which complaints resembling organic illnesses serve to mask neurotic disabilities.

XI. It has been pointed out that about 50 percent of all patients who consult civilian doctors are suffering basically from emotional problems. Yet our present system of medical school education allows only from 3 percent to 5 percent of the hours in the medical curriculum to orient the student in these problems. The absurdity in this situation is so obvious to anyone acquainted with it that we can only conclude we are dealing with either intellectual or emotional stupidity (it is probably the latter) on the part of our medical educators and university presidents. There is no other conclusion possible in terms of the size of the medical problem. By devoting more time to teaching psychiatry in the medical school curriculum, more physicians would become interested in it. As a matter of fact, the war experiences of physicians have convinced a rather large number of them that they should become trained and enter this specialty. Therefore, graduate and postgraduate training needs must be met and professional relationships improved if we are to approach the solution of the masses of psychiatric troubles that will continue to confront the nation and the world.

XII. Although attitudes are already changing slowly, one of the greatest tasks of all, and one that doctor and layman can share alike, is the education of the public to remove the almost universal fear and pessimism that exists about mental disorders. It is our duty to remove as soon as possible the popular misconceptions, some of which one hears expressed almost daily. I will mention only a few of these: Many people still believe that all psychiatric patients are crazy, noisy, destructive, and a danger either to themselves or others; that the patients are really all alike, varying only in degree of illness and dangerous potentialities; that people are either sane or insane; that mental illness starts suddenly when something "snaps" in the head or in one's mind; that a "nervous breakdown" is a disease of the brain or of the nerves; that most mental disorders are incurable; that you must always agree with a mentally ill person or you will get into a dangerous situation with him; that mental illness is a disgrace with immoral implications, or at least a lack of will power; and that it is a shame, a sign of inferiority, or a risk of being thought crazy to have to go to a psychiatrist. Because of these false convictions people postpone coming to the psychiatrist on their own behalf or sending their ill relatives until it is the last resort, and thus we receive the majority of our patients in a very ill condition, too often past psychiatric help.

XIII. Wars do teach us things but we all certainly would like to try to get along without them. Politicians still plan to end wars. Their activities and methods to that end are not very convincing. Repeated wars have certainly taught that if any politician, economist, or other specialist is now seeking a remedy to prevent wars, without utilizing the knowledge and techniques now available in the field of mental pathology, his efforts will be fruitless. Wars are basically the explosive expressions of mass emotional illnesses which have never been understood by those in a position to do something about it. To those who think deeply on these problems the outlook is usually foggy and dark, but sometimes Hope "sees a star" and "hears the rustle of a wing" that we trust belongs to the dove of peace hovering about seeking a place to roost, in safety from human aggression.

AMERICAN PIONEERING
IN PSYCHIATRY

By Howard W. Haggard, M.D.

FEW OF OUR greatest countrymen have ever brought about a more profound change in humanitarian ideology than did our countrywoman Dorothea Lynde Dix. She accomplished for the condition of the mentally ill of the world what Abraham Lincoln accomplished for the slaves of the United States. She was their emancipator.

But there is a fundamental difference in the two emancipations—a difference which carries with it a continuing responsibility. Slavery in our country ended with the freeing of one generation of slaves; it was entirely a social institution; it could be abolished completely by social change. But mental illness itself is not a social institution which can be ended by social reform. It is of each succeeding generation. Thus the accomplishment of Dorothea Dix was not an end but the beginning of a humanitarianism that must be kept alive and made to flourish in each generation. Although she died 60 years ago, she still lives in and with us and will continue to live in and with us as long as we cherish the ideology that she bequeathed to us.

Dorothea Lynde Dix is and was, I think, by any and every standard, the greatest woman our country, perhaps any country, has ever produced. And yet so little is she, her life, and her work, remembered by our public that she has become the "forgotten woman" of America. It is a curious commentary on our social values that when her name is mentioned the thoughts of most people turn not to a great emancipator who by a lifetime of toil and sacrifice added dignity and stature to our civilization, but instead to one whose fame has grown great among us from giving advice on sex and social problems to adolescents and chambermaids.

I say the last in no cynicism but, as you will see, with a practical, a utilitarian, idea in mind. Her lack of fame today can make no difference to Miss Dix. She had her vanities; but, so far as we can judge, a desire for posthumous fame was not one of them. Of the 32 hospitals for the care of the mentally ill which she founded in this country, she would permit only two to use a name even suggesting hers: Dix Hill in North Carolina and Dixmount in Pennsylvania, named after cities founded in Maine by her grandfather.

Fame during a lifetime is important in facilitating the accomplishment of missions. Miss Dix had that fame. She had ready admission to those of influence in many countries: high officials of our government and that of England received her, followed her advice, and welcomed her as a visitor to their homes. The Pope gave her a long and sympathetic audience. Deputations met her when her train, or river steamer, or stage coach stopped even in frontier towns. Railroads and steamship companies refused to charge her fares. In the War between the States she was in sole charge of organizing the nursing service of the Union Army. She held a rank in influence, if not by commission, defined as equal to that of a major general. At the close of hostilities the Secretary of War offered her any decorations and any honors that she would name. She named and accepted only one: a stand of arms of the colors of the United States. These flags hang today in the Memorial Hall of Harvard University and, bound in the archives, is a letter of commendation in terms superlative from Edwin Stanton, then Secretary of War. Yes, Miss Dix had, in her day, the fame and recognition that made easier the accomplishment of her difficult missions.

But, in contrast, her name is not mentioned in the contemporary medical histories of the Civil War. One can well understand that among those who provided the material for these histories, and among those who wrote them, there were resentments and antagonisms. Many a high-ranking officer lost argument and face to this woman who "intruded" into camp and hospital. There is little affection for those, no matter how good the intention and how beneficial the results, who outspokenly tell the world of our derelictions of duty, our inefficiencies, and our brutalities. And I wonder if perhaps the generations of us who came after Miss Dix have not unconsciously made the same reaction toward her work in exposing the inhumanities to the mentally ill that it is said the army historians made to her work in the nursing service. Perhaps a sense of guilt, and we may well have the guilt, has made its best defense in forgetting the name of Miss Dix, so that it fails to appear in our histories and schoolbooks and even in public knowledge.

One may speculate—and often speculate in elaborate error—but there is no speculation as to the fact that Miss Dix has been forgotten by a public that still needs her inspiration.

If I seem to have labored this point of fame it is for a purpose. Among our public, ideologies rarely persist, rarely flourish as abstractions; they must be supported by a personification that permits identification and emulation. At the simplest level the cherry tree and George Washington give to the child reality and comprehension of honesty that no abstraction could convey. At the highest level, religion gives us saintly lives to exemplify the virtues and thus serve as understandable and applicable demonstrations of principles. It is the lives of men and women that we understand —not ideologies. We set up leaders who exemplify the desirable qualities in human life and it is leaders—not ideologies—who permit emulation and identification.

The noble words of Lincoln carry their influence because behind them—in our sight, is the noble character of the man. The nursing profession gains in high principles because it has as its guiding influence the life, legend and symbolization of its saint—the Lady with the Lamp.

To the great loss of humanitarianism, Dorothea Dix, whose work was vastly more important than that of Florence Nightingale, never thus received lay canonization. Instead, she was forgotten; she was pushed from our minds. This loss is not a matter of historical injustice; it is one of profound practical importance; it bears directly on the regard in which today we hold the care of the mentally ill.

In my preamble, I have made strong claims that Miss Dix should be a national heroine. Let us together examine, with less emotion, the support of those claims and let us also, with no other excuse than human curiosity, peer into the make-up and the background of a great and good reformer.

First, the personal side. You can decide for yourself whether in her early life the weightier influence is heredity or environment. Both, for Miss Dix had peculiar elements. Her grandparents on her paternal side had exceptionally vigorous and unusual characters. Nothing is known about those on her maternal side, but the supposition is that they were less than remarkable. Her father, in spite of his superior heredity, was a ne'er-do-well, sometimes a convincing religious zealot and perhaps most often a drunkard. Her mother was an incompetent woman of little physical or moral vigor, eighteen years older than her husband.

The most striking ancestor was the grandfather, Elijah

Dix. He was born in 1747 of a "poor but upright" family in Watertown, Massachusetts. He apprenticed in medicine to Dr. John Green of Worcester, studied pharmacy under Dr. William Greenleaf in Boston, and set up in the practice of medicine in Worcester in 1770. A year later he married Dorothy Lynde of a prominent and wealthy family. Dr. Dix was successful in medicine but even more so in business. He speculated in Maine real estate, founding the towns of Dixmount and Dix Hill and he owned a fleet of vessels in the trade between New England and the West Indies. For wider fields of professional and business operations he moved to Boston in 1795. Dr. Dix was a man of violent and explosive temperament; he had many enemies; and, if stories may be trusted, he added generously to the number by his one recorded attempt at city reform. He wanted to have trees planted along the bare streets of Worcester but to the townspeople of that day and place a tree symbolized hardship— the hardship of clearing the land for farms. Bare places were beautiful. The suggestion and its author were unpopular.

Mrs. Dix, the paternal grandmother, was a woman of strong, upright and perhaps exacting character, but gentle and tactful in protecting her seven sons and one daughter from the unbridled tongue of their father. The third son, Joseph Dix, who was to become the father of Dorothea, was frail as a youth. He was compelled to leave Harvard—and virtually his family—because of his marriage, as an undergraduate, to Mary Bigelow whom his family considered ignorant, uncouth, and wholly undesirable. With his usual forthrightness, Dr. Dix relieved his responsibilities to his son, and at the same time removed him and his wife from Boston by settling him in Maine as agent for his land ventures there. The son and his wife lived in a log cabin in an unsettled country under conditions of extreme privation and hardship. Neither was equipped to meet this life. In the ill-kept cabin, to the complaining wife and the visionary —and often drunken husband—Dorothea was born in April, 1802. As a child, she played alone and thought alone and, to this fact she attributed an absorbing self-interest which she discovered in her young womanhood. One of the strongest driving forces of her adult life, and for her years of social reform, was the continual effort on her part to purge herself of this self-engrossment which, rightly or wrongly, she attributed to her childhood. We may have reservations as to the validity of her analysis of her own personality but of this we may be certain: as a child she was sorry for herself and her sorrow grew sharper when her position in the family was disturbed by the birth of two more children. Dorothea was without doubt a difficult child; she was also a determined one. At the age of twelve, whether with or without the consent of her parents, she left home and made the long trip to Boston alone to appeal to her grandmother to take her into her home and permit her to go to school in the city.

With the grandmother, who was punctilious in her desire to make the undisciplined child neat, punctual, respectful, and obedient, there were conflicts of personalities. There was a good deal of the iron of Grandfather Dix in Dorothea, but it was alloyed with self-pity and a sense of martyrdom. Hers, she thought—and said—was a life doomed to be loveless—no one cared for or wanted her.

After two years of the child, Grandmother Dix sent her to Worcester to board with an aunt. It was at Worcester that Dorothea, at the age of fourteen, opened a private school for small children. It is said that instead of profiting from her own experience as to the needs of childhood she was particularly severe, even for those days. Her discipline for little girls was that of humiliation; one child was compelled for a week to walk through the streets bearing a placard on her back with the legend: "A very bad girl, indeed."

After three years of teaching she returned to Boston, much improved, so it is said, in manners, habits, and neatness. She was, however, stubborn and headstrong and still self-interested. The grandmother, now seventy-one, was no match for the mental vigor of the girl. Dorothea ran the household. She opened a private school in the Boston home and, to the horror of her relatives, a small charity school for poor children as well. In addition, she embarked on a successful authorship of children's books. These activities kept her confined to her work from daybreak to well after midnight each day. One may wonder at this zeal for juvenile education in an adolescent, and one may speculate, perhaps fruitfully, as to what part of it was pathological: there was the strong driving force; there was the feeling of self-interest which must be uprooted; there was intense social timidity; and there was a love affair that began well, if timidly, that stiffened with overdemand and then ended suddenly with the quite normal young man marrying—I am sure to his best interests—not Dorothea, but a quite commonplace young lady.

The good Reverend William Ellery Channing, pastor of the church she attended, had an admiration and deep affection for Dorothea. He recognized her abilities and also her imperfections. For a time he took her into his family as tutor for his children and he counseled her long and kindly, inspiring her to an effort to rise above her imperfections and to meet and be a part of a broader life. At this stage her health failed with signs of active tuberculosis. A rest with the Channings at Saint Croix restored some measure of health and Dorothea, now thirty, returned to Boston determined to effect the change in her character which Dr. Channing had counseled.

I doubt much if this good man would have approved fully of the therapeutic regime she devised and instituted. I doubt also whether he appreciated the enormous driving force of her personality and the extent of her psychopathology. She again founded a school for the young and undertook to impart to the children the joy of self-mastery which she herself believed she was achieving. The secret of self-mastery, of moral and spiritual improvement, was zealous self-examination and introspection in order to find every fault and to remove it ruthlessly. It must have been, for the more impressionable children, a school for neuroses. If it were, they were soon spared, for the teacher's voice began to fail, hemorrhages came each day, the pain in her side was incessant. Finally, she could drive herself no more with castigation. She collapsed; and the school closed. The illness was long and severe. She went to England for convalescence. On her return to Boston, nearly two years later, she was frail in health and could no longer run a school. Her grandmother had died and left her a legacy sufficient to support her.

I have attempted—I trust not too unkindly—to outline the life of Miss Dix to the point where she was to commence her broad humanitarian work. If I have made her appear abnormal, let me add that abnormality of personality means only that she did not adjust well in an environment to which the majority of individuals adjusted best, and which is, for this reason, called a normal environment. The normal man —that is, the average man—does not desire radical changes in the fundamentals of his social environment, because they suit him as they are. The abnormal man may be broken by his maladjustment to the normal environment; only the exceptional one has the strength to break ties and traditions and to enter a new and radically different social environment. Miss Dix's personality did not alter as she aged—she grew in experience and diplomacy—but during the next forty years and more she created the environment to which her personality was suited, not the narrow confines of an elementary school, not sedentary study, not self-improvement by introspection, but the ruthless and bitter struggle to right a social injustice. To that task, she was bred and trained. And, the rarest of circumstances, she found, unaided, the opening in the walls that had imprisoned her during her earlier life.

The opening was a seemingly insignificant one; it came of chance and with no portent of its importance. It was simply this: a group of students of the Harvard Divinity School were assigned, for their experience, to Sunday School instruction in the East Cambridge jail. One of these young men was having little success with a class of some twenty female prisoners; he felt, I am sure wisely, that they should be led by a mature woman rather than a young man. He consulted his mother who, in turn, advised him to consult Miss Dix. The result was that on a Sunday in March, 1841, Miss Dix presented herself at the jail, her Bible under her arm, and her mind filled with thoughts of love and piety to be brought to unfortunate and repentant sinners. The sinners were unfortunate she found, but hardly repentant. It was her first experience with this phase of life—it was shocking. It was also challenging. The particular challenge, seemingly small at the time, concerned a number of mentally ill who, because there was no place else to house them, were thrust into jail. They were irresponsible of property, therefore their room was not heated with a stove; they were beasts, therefore they were not clothed; they were lunatics, therefore they had no physical or moral feelings to be satisfied by any kindly ministrations.

The challenge to Miss Dix that day was not the lofty one of humanitarianism for the mentally ill in general; it was only that the lunatics of the East Cambridge jail be given the same meager warmth, clothing, and food that the criminals of that prison had. She saw only a local injustice; it was only later, as she fought to correct a local illness, that she realized she was dealing with a disease of all society. As that realization came, her effort broadened from one jail in one town to the whole country and the whole world.

Before I deal with immediate events that grew from her Sunday in the East Cambridge jail, let me describe in a few words the attitude toward and the condition of the mentally ill in those days of the mid-nineteenth century.

The attitude toward and the care—or lack of care—accorded to the mentally ill has varied through the ages with the religious and social beliefs as to the causes of mental illness. By far the oldest and most persistent explanation for it was that of possession—possession by a spirit. Under some religious concepts—including nearly all pagan ones— possessing spirits might be either good or bad. The man possessed might, therefore, be revered as especially endowed: he was nearer to the spirits than the average man; and in his hallucinations he spoke to them or he spoke with their voice. He was to be respected, if only from fear of the spiritual consequences of ill treatment. Under Christian concept all possessing spirits were evil; they were demons not to be respected but to be exorcised. There grew up also a suspicion that the man or woman possessed had become so through some sin or by some deal of advantage with the forces of evil. If exorcism could not be readily effected by holy measures, there was an imputation of guilt. The victim of possession was therefore to be punished and punished cruelly—possibly even burned. This idea of partial personal responsibility for mental illness, or for its more violent manifestations, was to persist long after the idea of possession as a cause had been discarded. The consequence was restraint, and punishment, derision, and neglect.

Among physicians, the idea—expressed centuries earlier by Shakespeare—gradually developed that lunacy was a disease. Thus in the early nineteenth century Dr. Benjamin Rush—a great and influential figure in American medicine and one of the first of our physicians to write extensively on the diseases of the mind—advanced the theory that, and I quote, "madness is seated primarily in the blood vessels of the brain, and it depends upon the same kind of morbid and irregular action that constitutes other arterial diseases." However erroneous the pathology offered as a general causation, nevertheless it was a definite physical origin which would seem to bring madness into the category of any other physical disease and as deserving of the compassion awarded to the physical diseases. Rush further particularized the causes of the arterial disturbance to which he attributed madness as being abscesses, apoplexy, headache, alcohol, sex indulgence, extreme exercise, sudden changes of temperature, narcotics, consumption, skin eruption, and intense shock. Aside from sex, alcohol, and narcotics there was no element even suggesting depravity or volition in the causes. Further, Dr. Rush was one of the first American physicians to speak strongly for institutional care for the needy, as well as for the wealthy, mentally ill.

But no man, no matter how advanced his medical ideas may be, wholly escapes from the prevailing view of the society in which he is reared. Dr. Rush's therapy had in it elements suggesting strongly that the symptomatology of mental illness was not wholly due to a diseased condition in the arteries of the brain but arose from a maliciousness that needed to be subdued and disciplined. He bled his patients excessively and purged them mightily—a therapeutic mayhem that, in justice to him, he applied in most forms of illness. But for his mentally ill patients, in addition, he preserved a strict demeanor; he never laughed or talked with them; he believed that it was essential to be frigidly impersonal and dignified in dealing with them and that they should be controlled by fear. He used restraint; he employed, as "straighteners," exceedingly uncomfortable chairs in which the patients were bound; he whirled them in gyrators until they were stupefied with dizziness; he poured ice water over them; he threatened death; he starved them into submission; and he thought that pain was beneficial.

Rush was not interested in the humanitarian care of the mentally ill. I doubt if he regarded his patients as ill in behavior as well as ill in body. And I do not believe I do him an injustice in saying that his interest was solely that of a therapy for a physical pathology which he did not—and could not—comprehend as a cause of misbehavior. He believed, I think, that his patients misbehaved for the same reason that he conceived the drunk as misbehaving—simply from lack of restraint. Restraint, as he saw it, should be enforced.

Dr. Rush was a pioneer in the investigation of the medical treatment of mental illness. In this field he was far ahead of his day. But he did not realize that before advance in therapy could be made it was necessary to first have a new concept for the social, the humanitarian, regard in which the mentally ill were held.

The pioneer in that noble direction was a physician of France—Philippe Pinel. His work was done in the closing years of the eighteenth century. He was the physician in charge of a hospital, an institution of detention, for the mentally ill at Paris. There the inmates were manacled, chained in dungeons; they were beaten and starved. The mentally ill were guilty—guilty of God alone knows what—but guilty in the eyes of man. Pinel cut off the chains and manacles; he instituted a regimen of gentle, sympathetic, and humane care. There was no restraint, no discipline by force, and, constructively, there was occupational therapy to take the place of long hours, days, and years of idle brooding. The change in behavior of the patients was as radical as the change in care. Quietness and good behavior replaced shrieks and groans and violent struggles and brooding despair.

It was a propitious time for this revolution in care. Three years earlier the Bastille had fallen; the liberty of man was being proclaimed in France. The liberation of the inmates of the hospital was in keeping with the spirit of the French Revolution. Pinel was hailed as the "liberator of the insane."

However propitious its inception, this reform was overshadowed by the conflict of the French Revolution. But it was kept alive in England by the Quakers, through the efforts of William Tuke of York. Few things caused greater concern to the followers of this religion than the thought of their demented fellow members who were committed to the British workhouses. In 1792 Tuke, indignant over the treatment given in the York County Asylum, established the York Retreat with funds donated by Quakers. There, following Pinel's example, the mentally ill received decent quarters, good food, humane care, and medical treatment. It was the example of the Retreat and the vigorous action of the Quakers which, in England, led in 1840 to the elimination of restraint—manacles, chains and strait jackets—in the care of the mentally ill.

This step was not a complete one to the humane care of all mentally ill, but it was in the direction of removing the most striking barbarity. It was particularly notable in England, for that country has given our language an enduring word for the inhuman treatment of the mentally ill—the word "Bedlam." It is the English contraction of the word Bethlehem, the name of the great London prison asylum for madmen founded by Henry VIII in 1553 and for centuries one of the sights of the city. There, for sixpence, a man could take his family to see the madmen in chains; he, his wife and his children, could jeer and taunt the inmates until they shrieked and writhed in fury—and made the children laugh.

In the United States in 1840 what provision was made for indigent mentally ill—when any was made—was of three sorts: First, municipal, which in most instances consisted, as in East Cambridge at the time of the visit of Miss Dix, of prison facilities. The notable exceptions were good but small city institutions in Boston, New York, and Philadelphia. Second, there were county institutions, usually combined with poor farms. Sometimes the county care took the form of boarding out the mentally ill to the lowest bidders at public auctions. A farmer might attempt to make a profit out of lodging a mentally ill person in his barn or cellar for $1.25 to $2.00 a week. This county system led to the greatest of all abuses. In noting these sums I may say that $2.00 a week was $110 a year with money at a purchasing power far greater than today, perhaps four times greater. In this connection it was of interest to me to read in the daily press a few months ago that the figure given for the per capita cost of care of the mentally ill in the United States today was $400.

The third system, and the least developed in 1840, was that of state care. Eleven of the twenty-six states had made some appropriation of funds usually for the operation of a house of detention for mentally ill to relieve the jails. Usually no medical care was given, although in some states the inspiration for the erection of a state institution came, as it did in New York in 1836, from the state medical society. Hospitals such as the Massachusetts General which had a department for the care of the mentally ill (now the McLean Psychiatric Hospital), received little state or city support and depended upon legacies and donations. There were few private institutions and of these the most notable was the Hartford Retreat. Again a state medical society was instrumental in its founding and the financing of the institution is perhaps typical of the period. By private subscription $12,000 was raised; the state contributed $5,000 and the medical society $600. This total was augmented by $40,000 raised by a public lottery under state supervision.

In 1843 there were fourteen hospitals in the United States, private and public, devoted solely to the care of the mentally ill; their total bed capacity was 2,647. A commentary on the care given even a decade later is in the title of a paper read before a medical association of this country pleading "The Necessity of a Resident Medical Superintendent in an Institution for the Insane."

There were in the United States in 1840 a few citizens and some physicians who had enlightened and humane ideas regarding mental illness and the care of the mentally ill. But little progress could be made in providing suitable care until the ideas of the public at large became similarly enlightened and similarly humane. Any form of mental illness was regarded by the public as a disgrace; it was the hand of God—the sins of the father; it was the family skeleton to be closeted in deepest shame. Between the mentally ill and their own families a curtain of obscurity was dropped; only the pride of family and fear of censure made the members provide for their ill relations. These poor victims became prisoners, locked up if violent and hidden away if visitors approached the houses. Often they were imprisoned in a single room, perhaps manacled to the wall or bed. They were no longer human beings in the eyes of the family; no longer to be treated with friendly understanding, but instead they were either obviously humored or their wants and words were as obviously ignored. Now if men and women could, in the misfortune of disease, so regard and treat the members of their own family—parents, brothers, sisters, children—they could not regard and treat with higher understanding and humanity the strangers and the destitute who were mentally ill.

It was the labor of Dorothea Lynde Dix to bring that understanding to the public, and with it a desire for humane care, and to implant them so strongly that the public would do more than understand and hope—it would understand and pay. The change she wrought was not medical, it was social; she succeeded in making the public realize the relationship between social responsibility and taxation. She was that rarest of all human beings, one who made mankind more humane, who moved civilization toward the only valid advancement that civilization can make, humanitarianism, the correction of social injustice, the recognition of the brotherhood of man, and the acceptance of the privilege of participating in a higher civilization by some sacrifice of self. We are a better people because of this lonely, ill, and unhappy woman of Boston.

I make no claim that Miss Dix founded the humane care of the mentally ill; the principle was known long before her day, but principles alone brought no comfort to the mentally ill in prisons, cellars, and barns. She no more founded the principle of human care than did Florence Nightingale the principles of modern nursing. Those principles of nursing are described in the work of Paré, the surgeon who lived four hundred years before Miss Nightingale, and she herself learned them in a school open to female ex-convicts by the Lutheran Church. The tasks of Miss Nightingale and Miss Dix were primarily those of application.

There is a tendency, which I bewail and upon which I digress, but which we today are inclined to feel and show as a sort of snobbery: it is that discovery is more important than application. It is not. It only comes first. Without discovery there can be no application, but without application, discovery is barren; it bears no fruit.

The discovery of means to relieve human suffering, to promote health and abolish insecurity and to prevent untimely death (the essence of the only fundamental happiness that human beings may know) is and remains futile and academic until it is put into effect to accomplish these things. Application is to be respected as much as discovery—nay more, for when it involves social change it is more laborious and far less rewarding. The advancement of a civilization is not measured by what some few men know how to do but by what all men do. Miss Dix made this country great in the honor of the world. It is a shame we have forgotten her.

We return to Miss Dix as she leaves the East Cambridge House of Correction of a Sunday morning, indignant that the insane housed in that prison did not have the basic comforts given to the criminals. She was bent on correcting a local injustice. Miss Dix had no great difficulty in convincing the court that the mentally ill inmates should have better care; she was well supported in her local efforts by Horace Mann, Dr. Howe, and Charles Sumner—influential and humanitarian men of their day. The local condition was corrected, the mentally ill of the East Cambridge House of Correction had warmth and clothing, but the thoughts in her mind, the thoughts that would not let her rest, were: Is this a local condition? What are the conditions throughout Massachusetts? A few visits to neighboring towns showed her that those conditions were far more deplorable than any in the East Cambridge prison. She went to Howe and Mann and Sumner and asked them if the facts became known to the legislators of the state, would they respond for the larger and general situation as the courts of East Cambridge had responded for the lesser and specific situation? They gave as their opinion that they would. But they warned her that to present convincing evidence it would be necessary to obtain the facts at first hand.

It was from this conference that Miss Dix developed the pattern that guided her in all her future efforts in all parts of this country and in Europe. It consisted first in obtaining, on a large scale, undisputable evidence of brutality and neglect; second, of memorializing the legislatures with this evidence, and persistently putting upon them the burden of correcting a demonstrated, existing injustice. It was a method that worked. It worked first, because of the overwhelming mass of evidence that Miss Dix collected by her indefatiguable efforts; second, because of her tenacity in forcing the evidence before the eyes of the legislators; and third, because the people of the country were ready for a change. If Miss Dix had made her crusade fifty years earlier, I doubt that she would have succeeded; the people would not have been ready. But in those fifty years, social ideologies were becoming more humane. They were moving toward such demonstrations of humanitarianism as the principle of the common rights of all men, of the International Red Cross, and the abolition of slavery. Each of these movements needed only a leader to show the injustice, to point the way to remedy it—to give form and direction to the growing humanitarianism of the people. Miss Dix, for the mentally ill, showed an injustice, she pointed the way to correct it, and she opened the channel for a practical expression of a humanitarianism that existed but was latent and undirected in our people.

As I have said, she collected evidence. In Massachusetts, her first field, she traveled by horse and buggy, by stage coach to city, town and village. She visited jails, poor farms, cellars, attics and barns. In these she collected the material for what is possibly the most gruesome indictment of human neglect and cruelty ever to be published—her Memorial to the Legislature of Massachusetts. I quote a little of preamble and one or two of the situations described:

Gentlemen: I respectfully ask to present this material, believing that the cause, which actuates to and sanctions so unusual a movement, presents equivocal claim to public consideration and sympathy. Surrendering to calm and deep convictions of duty my habitual views of what is womanly and becoming, I proceed briefly to explain what has conducted me before you unsolicited and unsustained, trusting, while I do so, that the memorialist will be speedily forgotten in the memorial.

About two years since leisure afforded opportunity and duty prompted me to visit several prisons and almshouses in the vicinity of this metropolis. I found near Boston, in jails and asylums for the poor, a numerous class brought into unsuitable connection with criminals and the general mass of paupers. I refer to idiots and insane persons, dwelling in circumstances not only adverse to their own physical and moral improvement but productive of extreme disadvantage to all other persons brought into association with them. I applied myself diligently to trace the causes of these evils, and sought to supply remedies. Every new investigation has given depth to the conviction that it is only by decided, prompt and vigorous legislation that the evils to which I refer, to which I shall proceed more fully to illustrate, can be remedied. I shall be obliged to speak with great plainness, and to reveal many things revolting to the taste, from which my woman's nature shrinks with peculiar sensitiveness. I tell what I have seen. If I inflict pain upon you, and move you to horror, it is to acquaint you with sufferings which you have the power to alleviate, and make you hasten to the relief of the victims of legalized barbarity.

I come to present the strong claims of suffering humanity. I come to place before the Legislature of Massachusetts the

conditions of the miserable, the desolate, the outcast. I come as
the advocate of helpless, forgotten insane, and the idiotic men
and women; of being sunk to a condition from which the most
unconcerned would start with real horror.

. . . The condition of human beings, reduced to the extrem-
est states of degradation and misery, cannot be exhibited in
softened language, or adorn a polished page.

I proceed, gentlemen, briefly to call your attention to the
present state of insane persons confined within this Common-
wealth, in cages, closets, cellars, stalls, pens. Chained, naked,
beaten with rods, and lashed into obedience.

As I state cold, severe facts, I feel obliged to refer to persons
and definitely to indicate localities.

I may say, parenthetically, that the only florid language
in the whole Memorial was in this preamble. The language
of the body of the Memorial describing what she saw was so
restrained, so barren of detail as to intensify the horror of it.
I quote only two instances:

Danvers. November. Visited the almshouse. Here 56 to 60 inmates, one idiotic, 3 insane. Found the mistress and was conducted to a low building rather remote from the principal
building; here a young woman exhibiting a condition of neglect and misery blotting out the faintest idea of comfort. She
had been, I learned, a respectable person, industrious and
worthy. She became a maniac. She had been at Worcester Hospital for a time and had been returned as incurable. While
there she was said to be decent. There she stood now, clinging
to or beating upon the bars of her caged apartment, the con-
tracted size of which afforded space only for increasing accumu-
lation of filth. There she stood with naked arms and disheveled
hair, the unwashed frame invested with fragments of unclean
garments, the odor so extensively offensive that it was not possible to remain beyond a few moments. Irritation of the body,
produced by utter filth and exposure, incited her to the horrid
process of tearing off her skin. Her face, neck and person were
thus disfigured to hideousness. She held up a fragment just rent
off. To my exclamation of horror the mistress replied: "Oh, we
can't help. We can do nothing with her; and it makes no dif-

ference what she eats, for she consumes her own filth as readily as the food which is brought her."

Newton: Over the woodshed. Unheated. Furniture a wooden box with straw and something I was told was a man half buried in the offensive mass. Protruding from the foot of the box were stumps and to these maimed members, were swinging chains, fastened to the side of the building. The master of the house briefly stated the history of the wretched victim. As, till within a late period the town had owned no farms for the poor, this man with others had annually been put up at auction. And a few winters since, being kept in an outhouse, the people within, being warmed and clothed, did not reckon on how cold it was and so his feet were froze. He cannot now walk or run. But he was chained. He might crawl forth and do some harm.

These are not extreme instances I have chosen from the Memorial. To me, far more chilling in her writings are often single statements that tell a horror. Thus a sentence in which the wife of the keeper of the almshouse said of an old man "he's quieter now since the last time my husband went in and tamed him."

The Memorial was presented to the legislators. It was vigorously denied by the men of the towns named. It was supported and verified by prominent citizens and physicians who rallied to the aid of Miss Dix. The money was appropriated to enlarge the state facilities for the care of the mentally ill. The procession of sad victims started from cellars, dens, barns, closets, prisons, and almshouses to new, clean quarters where they would be treated kindly, fed, and sheltered—aided when medicine could aid them—and given what was the supreme consolation, that of being treated by human beings as human beings.

The rest of Miss Dix's life was mainly the repetition under greater hardship and with unremitting effort, night and day, of the work she had done in Massachusetts. Rhode Island, Connecticut, and New York increased their facilities.

New Jersey had no state care, and when the Legislature, after the delays and protests that followed her Memorial, built the great institution at Trenton, it was to her, her first-born child. It was the beginning of a large family that grew state by state and country by country.

It is said she obtained larger appropriations of money for benevolent purposes than probably was ever given any mortal to raise. But in the effort to obtain these appropriations there came the greatest disappointment of her life. For six years she had appealed to the United States Congress to lay aside federal lands for the support of the nation's hospitals for the mentally ill. For two years she lived in Washington, working day and night, summer and winter, to get the bill supported. At the end of this time the bill was passed by both Houses. It was vetoed by President Pierce.

To Miss Dix, her efforts in organizing and heading the nursing service in the War between the States was only an incident in a lifetime of unremitting public service, as was her work in relief at the Chicago fire in 1871 and that of Boston in 1872, and the raising of funds for the monument which she designed to the fallen soldiers at the National Cemetery at Hampton, Virginia. These were minor to the great accomplishment which is marked by thirty-two American state institutions erected solely by her efforts—institutions in which there could ever after be demonstrated and measured the level of humanitarianism of this country.

I have said little of the life of Miss Dix after the days of her Memorial to the Legislature of Massachusetts. And if I have been terse here, I want to be more so in summing up her life. I can only hope that my two sentences will carry to you the conviction that the words in her Memorials carried to the people of her day. My words are these: Dorothea Lynde Dix was the greatest woman this country, perhaps any country, has ever produced. If we prescribe to the belief that the basis of civilization is humanitarianism, then she deserves to be brought out of the oblivion that now surrounds her memory and take her place as our national heroine.

ANTI-INFECTIOUS AGENTS
OF NATURAL ORIGIN

The George R. Siedenburg Memorial Lecture

By René J. Dubos, Ph.D.

FOR THE third time in seven years, one of the Lectures to the Laity of The New York Academy of Medicine is devoted to the problem of the chemotherapy of infectious diseases. Two former contributors to the series, Drs. Perrin H. Long and Colin MacLeod, directed much of their attention to the study of those drugs—the sulfonamides in particular—which are prepared synthetically in the chemical laboratory. I shall here deal more specifically with another type of drugs, not synthetic preparations of the chemist, but on the contrary natural products extracted from biological materials, and especially from microorganisms. Penicillin is today the most famous of the latter group of chemotherapeutic agents.

When Dr. Long wrote his paper in 1940, the curative activity of sulfanilamide had been recognized for only a few years. The new sulfa drugs, sulfapyradine and sulfathiazole, had just been announced. For the first time, streptococcus septicemia, pneumococcus pneumonia, cerebrospinal meningitis, gonorrhea, etc., had become amenable to treatment with synthetic drugs. All could agree with the 1940 lecturer that we had reached the era of "Chemical warfare against disease."

In 1940, Dr. MacLeod entitled his contribution "The Past, Present, and Future of chemotherapy." The predictions made three years earlier by Dr. Long had been fully verified. Sulfadiazine and other highly useful synthetic derivatives of sulfanilamide had been added to the family of sulfa drugs. Moreover, much had been learned of the mechanism of action of the new wonder drugs, and this knowledge suggested a rational methodology for the synthesis of other types of chemotherapeutic agents. The time had come when one could, almost at will, devise new types of substances capable of interfering with the living processes of any microbial agent and consequently of inhibiting its multiplication.

Although the chemical approach to the warfare against disease was thus fulfilling all hopes, Dr. MacLeod found it necessary to remind his audience that the ancient pharmacopeia was composed entirely of remedies of plant origin. Even today some of these plant remedies have retained an essential place in the treatment of certain parasitic infections; for example, the quinine used in the treatment of malaria is extracted from the bark of the cinchona tree, and emetine, still the most effective drug for amoebic dysentery, is an alkaloid crystallized from the ipecacuanha root. The curative properties of these plant products, both of them native to South America, had been recognized by the native populations long before European physicians adopted them into the pharmacopeia. In fact, it was several centuries before chemists established the nature of the active chemical principle of the plant extracts, and before parasitologists identified the microbial parasites against which the treatment was directed. There was an obvious reason for this renewal of interest in biological materials as sources of useful drugs. Two new substances, penicillin and gramicidin, had just been shown capable of controlling certain types of infectious diseases—and both these substances had been extracted from microorganisms, one from the culture of a mold, the other from a culture of a bacterium, in other words from the lowest representatives of the plant kingdom.

During the immediately following years, the search for anti-microbial agents produced by microorganisms was to become one of the most lively fields of occupation of the microbiologist. Fads and fashions affect the activity of men of science as they govern the games and gossip of the drawing room or the shape of women's hats. During the late 1930s, chemists and bacteriologists were busy synthesizing in the laboratory or testing in animals thousands of new derivatives of sulfonamides. In the early 1940s, fashion had changed and the search for antimicrobial agents of biological origin had become the favorite indoor sport of many biologists. All over the world thousands of types of bacteria, actinomycetes, molds, higher fungi, algae, plants (their bark, their leaves, their flowers and their fruits), animals (their tissues and products) have been extracted with neutral, acid, or alkaline water, with alcohol, acetone, ether, and every conceivable solvent, in the hope of discovering some new drug useful in the treatment of infectious disease. It is too early to evaluate the fruits of this frantic activity, but it is obvious that nothing comparable to penicillin has as yet been discovered. It is true that there have been found many hundreds and probably thousands of new substances capable of killing bacteria and other parasites or of inhibiting their growth in the test tube. But among the many substances which are bactericidal or bacteriostatic *in vitro* (to use the lingo of the bacteriologist), only very few are proving useful in the treatment of disease and can qualify as chemotherapeutic agents.

This extraordinary contrast between ordinary antiseptic activity (active only outside of the body) and chemotherapeutic usefulness (effective in the treatment of disease) is not a new experience for the student of infection. Immediately after the recognition of microbes as agents of disease, it was discovered that many common substances of known chemical structure exhibit a powerful inhibitory and even a killing effect on many infectious agents. Thus chlorine and iodine and their derivatives, mercury and all the various organic mercurials, carbolic acid and many other coal-tar products, different types of soap or like substances, hydrogen peroxide, and so on and so on, have long been known to possess powerful antiseptic or germicidal properties. It soon became obvious, however, that most anti-microbial substances are useless or even objectionable in the treatment of disease, for two reasons. On the one hand, many of them lose their germicidal activity in the presence of animal tissues because the latter contain substances which react with the antiseptic and inhibit its antimicrobial action; on the other hand, practically all of them are more toxic for tissue cells than for the parasites responsible for infection. The experience of half a century of organic chemistry applied to the discovery of anti-microbial substances has emphatically shown that it is as easy to synthesize new powerful antiseptics, as it is difficult to discover one which can be used in the treatment of infection.

Prior to 1935 there were many indeed who felt that the search for chemotherapeutic agents effective in the body against bacterial infections was a hopeless venture. The statement made by Von Behring in the 1880s still expressed the general point of view of most students of infectious disease:

It can be regarded almost as a law that the tissue cells of man and animal are many times more susceptible to the poisonous effects of disinfectant than any bacteria known at present. Before the antiseptic has a chance either to kill or inhibit the growth of the bacteria in the blood or in the organs of the body, the infected animal itself will be killed. Therefore the pessimism of him who declared that disinfection in the living body is for all time impossible appears to be only too justified.

In this light it becomes easier to evaluate the great importance for the history of chemotherapy of the recognition that sulfonamides are effective curative agents. In the test tube, sulfonamides are less powerful than chlorine, mercuric chloride, hydrogen peroxide, or many common antiseptics, but unlike these substances they have the remarkable property of possessing only limited toxicity for the human body, and of retaining their activity in the presence of living tissues.

The contrast between an ordinary antiseptic and a chemotherapeutic agent is equally striking when examples are selected among substances extracted from animal, plant, or microbial cells. Plants, for example, produce a great variety of powerful antiseptics; we may mention among many others the substance responsible for the pungent odor of garlic, some of the essential oils extracted from flowers, some of the soap-like material known as saponins. But few are the plant products which are useful in the treatment of infection; quinine and emetine have already been mentioned.

The fact that microorganisms can produce substances inhibitory to other microorganisms was also recognized very early. In fact, it is interesting to note that recognition of the existence of anti-microbial agents of biological origin dates from the very beginning of microbiology. In his very first paper on the microbial theory of fermentation, Pasteur remarked that onion juice contains a substance—probably an essential oil—which inhibits the production of alcohol by yeast, and also prevents the growth of certain protozoa. A few years later he observed furthermore that certain saprophytic free-living germs, present in soil and in the air, destroyed the virulence of cultures of anthrax bacilli, and he ventured to state, "These facts perhaps justify the highest hopes for therapeutics."

It would be impossible, and indeed useless, to review once more the many examples of inhibition of pathogenic micro-organisms by products of biological origin which have been described during the past 75 years, and the attempts which have been made to apply these findings to the treatment of disease. Suffice it to say that most of these products suffer from the limitations already mentioned in the case of anti-septics of chemical origin; they lose most of their antimicrobial activity in the presence of animal tissues; they are toxic for the human body. Of all substances known, only one so far has proved free or almost free from these objections, namely the product of the mold *Penicillium notatum,* which has achieved fame under the name of penicillin. So many have spoken of its miraculous virtues that to recite them again appears a waste of your time. In fact, a recent statement by Sir Howard Florey, an Australian by birth, appears worth quoting at this time:

So much has been written and talked about penicillin, that I feel I am in danger of becoming like some other Australian birds—they sing perfectly a short series of notes, but repeat them so often that they become rather boring. So today I thought it might be more interesting to put before you an account of some of the work on the use in medicine of naturally occurring antibacterial substances. There are still many misapprehensions on this subject, and it is one of the fields in which some historical information is of help in the orientation of one's ideas at the present time.

I would like then, not to try to imitate the sweet song of the Australian bird, but to discuss instead some of the difficulties and pitfalls which make it unlikely that many other miraculous penicillin-like substances will be found in nature. To date only three substances of microbiological ori-

gin—penicillin, streptomycin, and gramicidin—have been
sufficiently studied to permit accurate evaluation of their
properties, merits, and limitations. I shall attempt to discuss the characteristics of these three substances in order to
illustrate some of the factors which have to be taken into
account for the evaluation of a new antibacterial drug.

Penicillin. It has been recently established that penicillin is a generic name for a family of substances (penicillins
K, F, G, X, etc.) all produced by the mold *Penicillium
notatum.* Although all these penicillins exhibit approximately the same antibacterial activity in the test tube, they
differ appreciably in their ability to control disease in the
human and animal body. Much higher doses of penicillin
K than of penicillin G or X, for example, are required for
the same therapeutic effect; it appears likely at the present
time that this difference is due to the fact that penicillin K
reacts much more avidly than the other penicillins with
certain constituents of the blood, and therefore becomes
unavailable for antibacterial activity. These facts illustrate the advisability of utilizing preparations of the drug
of known purity in order to obtain reproducible results in
clinical practice. Fortunately, commercial preparations of
crystalline penicillin of a high degree of purity are now available. These preparations are remarkably free of toxic properties and—except in the case of a few individuals exhibiting
peculiar idiosyncrasies—can be safely injected into the human body in enormous amounts.

Let us now consider the few limitations of this miraculous
substance. Unfortunately, it is rapidly destroyed in the
stomach, a fact which limits its administration in the form of
pills or tablets and renders necessary more cumbersome
methods of injection. Furthermore, penicillin is rapidly
eliminated from the body in the urine. In order to maintain
adequate therapeutic concentrations in the body fluids, it is

sometimes necessary to keep on injecting the drug at short intervals of time. These practical defects are only of little significance and can be overcome by the skill of the physician; they do emphasize, however, that the maximal effectiveness of a drug can be achieved only on the basis of accurate knowledge of the multiple factors—rates of adsorption, destruction, and excretion—which control its concentration in the body.

Of more fundamental importance is the fact that penicillin is not equally active against all types of infectious agents. Some, like the germs of tuberculosis, typhoid, and whooping cough, or like the viruses which cause influenza, the common cold, measles, and other diseases are resistant to it. Moreover, the different strains within a given bacterial group often vary greatly in their susceptibility. Thus, among the staphylococci found in many types of abcesses, or among the streptococci which cause disease of the heart valves, many are highly susceptible to the drug, and some much more resistant. It is unreasonable, therefore, and indeed objectionable, to use penicillin indiscriminately for any and every infectious ailment. Ideally, it would be desirable— but unfortunately not always practical—to determine beforehand the susceptibility to the drug of the causative agent of the disease, in order to establish therapy on rational ground.

Streptomycin. Streptomycin is produced by *Actinomyces griseus,* a filamentous microorganism, smaller than the ordinary molds, but larger than bacteria. Among the many valuable characteristics of this interesting substance is the fact that it inhibits several of the bacterial species which are not affected by penicillin, among them the germs of tuberculosis, rabbit fever (tularemia), whooping cough.

Although streptomycin is one of the least toxic chemotherapeutic agents, it is not entirely an innocuous substance.

Repeated injections of doses exceeding 2 to 3 grams daily cause in particular some injury to the 8th cranial nerve, with consequent impairment of hearing and other functions. In the case of diseases which, like tularemia or certain types of infection of the urinary tract, respond rapidly to streptomycin therapy, the potential toxicity of the drug is only a minor factor. However, the problem of toxicity becomes much more important in the treatment of tuberculosis, for a number of independent reasons which we shall attempt to analyze presently.

Tuberculosis is characterized by multiple centers of infection, in which the germ is often protected by tissue barriers against the action of antibacterial agents; furthermore, although streptomycin has a marked inhibitory effect on the multiplication of the tubercle bacillus, it is much less effective in killing this organism and therefore in completely ridding the body of infection. For these two reasons, it is necessary to maintain high concentrations of the drug in the blood stream during prolonged periods of time, in order to achieve a significant therapeutic effect. The physician consequently often resorts to the difficult technique of repeated injections several times daily in order to repress the growth of the bacillus and permit the body to overcome the infection. Needless to say, these are the very conditions under which toxic manifestations of the drug become most evident and too often interfere with successful therapy.

The failure to eradicate completely and rapidly the tuberculous infection has other very serious consequences. It is well known that, as a result of exposure to sublethal concentrations of a given drug, bacterial cultures can give rise by adaptation and selection to variant forms which are still capable of producing disease, but which have become highly resistant to the drug. To use a striking if not highly accurate terminology, tubercle bacilli can be *trained* to become resistant to streptomycin. Thus tuberculous patients in which the disease has been arrested by streptomycin treatment often exhibit a relapse of the infection, caused by a drug-resistant form of the tubercle bacillus which is no longer amenable to streptomycin therapy.

On account of the chronicity and peculiar pathology of tuberculosis, due to the existence of centers of infection in which the bacilli are protected by tissue barriers, the tubercle bacillus lends itself readily to the production and demonstration of drug resistance. The phenomenon, however, is not peculiar to the tubercle bacillus and streptomycin. It has been observed in numerous types of experimental and natural infections, with many types of drugs. Indeed, it is commonly observed wherever therapy has not been adequate to achieve rapid and complete sterilization of the infectious process; that is, under conditions in which the microorganism persists for prolonged periods of time in contact with concentrations of the drug that are effective in repressing bacterial growth but not sufficient to exert a completely killing effect on the bacteria.

Gramicidin. Whereas penicillin is produced by a mold and streptomycin by an actinomycete, gramicidin is extracted from an even smaller type of microorganism, a bacillus commonly found in nature, *Bacillus brevis.* Gramicidin can be readily prepared in the pure crystalline state; however, it has been used most often in the form of a less purified alcoholic extract of *Bacillus brevis,* known as tyrothricin. It exhibits a high degree of activity against a number of virulent bacteria, in general the same which are susceptible to penicillin, and is inactive against many of the germs which are resistant to the latter substance.

Gramicidin is extremely stable under all sorts of conditions and is readily prepared at a fairly low cost. Its antibacterial activity is not markedly decreased in the presence of blood plasma and moreover its killing effect on susceptible bacteria is more rapid than that of penicillin and streptomycin. Finally, it is innocuous for certain types of tissue cells, for example for the white corpuscles of the blood. One might anticipate that these valuable properties would render gramicidin a very useful chemotherapeutic agent. It becomes of special interest for our discussion, therefore, to inquire why this drug cannot occupy a place comparable to that of penicillin in the treatment of infectious diseases. One reason is that gramicidin is poorly soluble in water and consequently does not reach a satisfactory distribution in infected tissues. More important is the fact that this drug, although devoid of toxicity for certain types of tissue cells, is a violent poison for other types, causing, for example, the dissolution of red blood cells. Injection of gramicidin into the blood stream brings forth severe toxic reactions which preclude its utilization in the treatment of systemic infections even in cases where the causative microorganism is extremely susceptible to the drug.

With adequate understanding of the great limitations of gramicidin, it becomes possible to select a few diseases where it can exert its anti-bacterial action without manifesting any toxic effect. Thus bovine mastitis, an infection localized in the udder of dairy cows, can be treated successfully by injecting gramicidin (or tyrothricin) directly into the infected udder. The drug is also used in human medicine for the treatment of certain superficial infections, for example of leg ulcers. In these two cases (bovine mastitis and superficial ulcers), gramicidin is brought directly into contact with the surface infection and can exert its anti-bacterial effect; because of its insolubility, on the other hand, it has no opportunity to reach the blood stream where it could cause destruction of red blood cells and other toxic reactions. These, obviously, are narrow conditions of usefulness. We have cited this example to illustrate the fact that reports of successful clinical results with a given drug in certain specified pathological conditions are not in themselves adequate basis for hope of similar success in other diseases.

Penicillin, streptomycin, and gramicidin have been selected for discussion because they permit an analysis of some of the many factors which condition the usefulness of an antibacterial substance in clinical practice.

Other drugs—including subtilin, and bacitracin—also extracted from cultures of saprophytic microorganisms, have been described more recently and may soon become available; they will demand extensive and complex clinical trials before their merits and limitations are properly defined. It will be necessary to determine in each case the acute and chronic toxicity of the new substances; the rates at which they are absorbed, modified, destroyed, and excreted in the human body; the ranges of microorganisms which they attack; whether they only inhibit their growth or actually exert a killing effect on them; how readily and completely the susceptible microorganisms develop resistance to the drug, and therefore how permanent is its therapeutic effect. These are only some of the many properties and reactions that remain to be ascertained.

Against this complex background, it becomes easier to appreciate that the discovery of a new agent which exhibits antibacterial effect in the test tube has only little significance for the student of infection; it is only the first and simplest in a long series of steps which are required to define the therapeutic value of a substance. Of the many "miracle germ killing substances" which are announced in your morning newspaper or in your favorite magazine, very few will cure a mouse of an experimental infection, still fewer will ever reach the office of your physician. For a long time to come, it appears, penicillin will remain the glamor girl among anti-infectious agents of microbial origin.

It has become obvious that the theoretical and practical problems of chemotherapy are identical, whether the drug under consideration is, like the sulfonamides, synthesized in the chemical laboratory, or, like quinine, extracted from the bark of a tree, or produced by a mold as in the case of penicillin. The origin of a substance is of no significance with reference to its clinical usefulness, indeed of no significance with reference to any of its properties. Thus quinine was first extracted from a plant, but it can also be synthesized in the chemical laboratory now that its molecular structure has been established. Similarly the chemist can break apart and inactivate the penicillin produced by the mold, then determine its structure, finally reconstitute it by synthesis in the original active form. It may be objected that the chemical syntheses of quinine or penicillin do not have as yet practical possibilities; this objection is of no importance for the theory and practice of chemotherapy; only comparative costs of production will decide whether penicillin is prepared by chemical synthesis from coal-tar derivatives, or extracted from cultures of the mold grown in millions of gallons of a broth consisting of corn-steep liquor and milk sugar. The natural produce of today may become the synthetic chemical of tomorrow; and penicillin will be the same substance, exhibit the same properties, and present the same biological problems, whether its origin is natural or synthetic.

As appears from the history of antisepsis and chemotherapy, it is easy to discover new substances endowed with anti-microbial activities *in vitro,* but most unusual to find one which is useful in the treatment of disease. The chemist is beginning to recognize a few generalizations—a few correlations between molecular structure and therapeutic activity—which guide him in the search for desirable properties in synthetic compounds. On the contrary, the biologist extracting plant tissues or microbial cultures, proceeds empirically, blindly, by hit and miss, spurred on by the hope that he will again find on his way some other penicillin-like wonder drug. Nevertheless, the hunt among living things has not been unproductive, despite its empirical character. Not only has it yielded a few substances of proved or possible therapeutic value; it has simultaneously revealed new types of chemical structures associated with biological activity which would have remained unsuspected otherwise. The physician marvels at the anti-infectious activity of penicillin; but the chemist also discovers with surprise a type of molecular constitution which he had not anticipated. Likewise, the biochemist and the biologist, as they analyze the mechanism of action of the drug, are now hoping to recognize unexpected ways of interfering with the processes of microbial life. Similarly, gramicidin and streptomycin are revealing types of chemical structure and of biological activity which were unavailable heretofore. Thus a few new pages of the Great Book of Nature are being deciphered, unfolding new combinations of molecular arrangement and of active properties which man had not known, or dared to conceive. When removed from direct contact with the world of natural objects, the imagination of the scientist, like that of the artist, becomes sterile, or at least sluggish. The search for anti-infectious agents in the realm of living things will be fruitful in opening new paths of investigation and suggesting new lines of endeavor, even if it does not yield another penicillin. Following the era of exploration, should come that of exploitation and more rational development. As he unravels the chemical nature of the natural products, and the structural determinants of their biological activity, man will soon learn to reproduce them at will, then to improve upon them.

A devout nineteenth century English parson, convinced that the Almighty in his kindness had placed a remedy near the source of all suffering, prepared from the willow—a tree of the wet lowlands—an extract which eased the rheumatic pains so frequent among the inhabitants of damp countries. Even the most humble peasant woman has now forgotten the medicinal virtues of the willow extract and uses, instead, aspirin produced from coal-tar in the chemical factory. Aspirin, says the chemical dictionary, is acetyl salicylic acid. Salicylic acid? The word comes from *Salix,* the Latin name of the willow tree. The chemist has determined the molecular structure of the active principle of the plant extract and, after learning to synthesize it in his laboratory, has preserved in the name the origin of his discovery. By modifying salicylic acid, he then improved on nature to produce aspirin. This passage from willow extract to aspirin symbolizes the evolution of chemotherapy; few now are those who remember the devout English parson and the humble willow.

The powerful and mysterious substances which the biologist extracts from living things excite today wonder and awe; their chemical formulas will be a matter of course in the textbooks of tomorrow; and the physician himself will have forgotten their origin when these substances appear in a hundred modified forms in the pharmacopeia of next year.

INDEX

Amputees, care of, 13 f.

Anti-infectious agents, 92 ff.

Anti-microbial substances, objections to some, in the treatment of disease, 95

Antiseptics, limitations as germicidal agents, 95

Army, physical examination, 5 f.; vaccination and immunization vs. disease, 8; casualties, 11; surgical care, 11 ff.; evacuation and treatment of wounded, 12 ff.; rehabilitation program, 16 f.; discharges for personality disorders, 56; common neurotic reactions, 57 f.

—— Medical Department, services in World War II, 5 ff.

Army General Classification Test, 61 f.

Aspirin, relation to willow extract, 106

Atabrine, 7 f.

Atom, medical use of, 18 ff.; research, 32 ff.

Atomic Energy Commission, 29

"Baby sitter," 52

Bakwin, Harry, 47

"Bedlam," 82

Behring, Emil A. von, quoted 95 f.

Bender, Lauretta, 47

Bigelow, Mary, 73

Bingham, W. V., "Inequalities in Adult Capacities: from Military Data," 62

Blind, the, care of, 13

"Breaking point" of the individual under stress, 58

Bunnell, Sterling, 14

Carbon, 11, 14, 35, 36

Chadwick, Sir James, 21 f.

Channing, William Ellery, 75

Chemotherapy of infectious diseases, 92 ff.

Child care, 37 ff.; methods of, 38 ff.; investigation and research in, 40; working mothers and, 41; "Nursery" vs. "Foundlinghome," 47 ff.; "baby sitters," 52

Children, need for affection, 41 ff.; rearing of, in modern society, 43 f.; effect of separation from mothers, 45 ff.

Civilians, psychiatric stresses in wartime, 55 ff.; wartime neuroses, 59

Civil War, services of Dorothea Dix, 70 f.

Clinics, need for, 65

Conant, James B., 34 f.

Curie, Irène, *see* Joliot-Curie

Cyclotron, 31

DDT, 8

Deaf, the, 15

Dentistry, services of the profession to the Army, 16

Dix, Dorothea Lynde, life and career, 69 ff.; Memorial to the Legislature of Massachusetts, quoted, 87 ff.

Dix, Elijah, 72 f.

Electric shock treatment, 10

Emetine, 93

Erpf, Stanley F., 9

Farrand, Livingston, 4

Fat, research on behavior of, in the body, 34 ff.

Fermi, E., 22
Florey, Sir Howard, quoted, 97
Foreign-body locator, 10
"Foundlinghome" vs. "Nursery," 47 ff.

Goldfarb, Walter, 47
Gramicidin, 93, 105; description and limitations of, 102 ff.
Green, John, 73
Greenleaf, William, 73
"Group Psychotherapy," 64

Half-life, disintegration of radioactive elements, 20 f., 24
Helium, 19 f.
Hevesy, Georg, 24
Hospitals, general, availability for psychiatric patients, 66
Hospitals, psychiatric, needed improvements in, 64 f.
Howe, Samuel Gridley, 85
Hypnosis, psychotherapeutic use of, 63 f.

Individual, the, predisposition to neuroses, 57, 60 f.
Infants, research in emotional development of, 44; findings, 45 f.
Infectious diseases, chemotherapy of, 92 ff.
Influenza, vaccine vs., 9
Iodine, radioactive, 27 ff.

Joliot-Curie, Frédéric and Irène, 18, 18 f.; demonstration of artificial radioactivity, 21 ff.

Kilogram, international, 20

Lawrence, Ernest, 23, 31
Leukemia, chronic myelogenous, 25 f.
Linsly, William R., career, 3 f.
Long, Perrin H., 92
Lowrey, Lawson G., 47

MacLeod, Colin, 92 f.
Malaria, use of atabrine vs., 7 f.

Mann, Horace, 85
Mentally ill, historic reactions toward, 78 ff.
Microorganisms, anti-microbial agents produced by, 92 ff.
Moorhead, Dr., 10
Mothers, working, and child care, 41
Mothers, training of, 49 ff.
"Mother substitute," 47

"Narcosynthis," 63
National Research Council, services in World War II, 7 ff.
Neuroses, individual predisposition to, 57, 60 f.
Neurosurgical cases, care and treatment of, 14 f.
Neutron, discovery of, 21
New York Academy of Medicine, founding, and work of, 37 f.
"Nursery" vs. "Foundlinghome," 47 ff.

Overindulgence, of children, 42

Paré, Ambroise, 84
Penicillin, 7, 10, 93, 104, 105; Florey quoted *re*, 97; description and limitations of, 98 f.
Phosphorus, radioactive, 24 f.; as a tracer element, 32
Physicians, the general practitioner and psychiatry, 66
Pinel, Philippe, services to the mentally ill, 80 f.
Plasma, 9 f.
Plastic surgery, 15
Polycythemia vera, 26 f.
Porter, William C., 60
Psychiatry, problems and services of, in wartime, 54 ff.; teaching of, and the general practitioner, 66 f.; public education in, 67
Psychoneuroses, wartime, therapeutic procedures, 55, 59; diagnostic labels for, 57; therapeutic procedures, 58 f.

Psychosis, treatment of, 10
Psychotherapeutic techniques, 63

Quinine, 93, 104

Radioactive elements, research in, and medical application of, 18 ff.; half-life, 20 ff.; as tracers, 29
Radioactivity, discoveries of Irène and Frédéric Joliot, 18 ff.; artificial, discovery of, 21 ff.; medical role of, 24
Radium, half-life, 20 f.
Rayleigh, Lord, 20
Rehabilitation, 16 f.; *see also* Psychotherapeutic techniques
Rhoads, C. P., 24*n*; quoted, 28
Rorschach test, 62f.
Rush, Benjamin, *re* mental illness, 79 f.
Rutherford, Lord, 21

Schistosomiasis, 15
Schoenheimer, Rudolf, 33 f.
Selective Service, rejections for personality disorders, 56
Shock treatment, 63
Sodium pentothal, psychotherapeutic use of, 63
Strecker, Edward A., 51
Sulfa drugs, 10
Streptomycin, 7, 105; description and limitations of, 99 f.
Sulfa drugs, 92 f., 96
Sumner, Charles, 85

Tantalum, 10
Tests, psychologic, as diagnostic aids, 61 ff.
Thatcher, John S., 3
Thyroid cancer, 27 f.
Tracer elements, 32
Tuberculosis, and streptomycin, 100 f.
Tuke, William, York Retreat, 81
Tunisia, British Army rehabilitation program, 16
Typhus, 8

United States, 19th century provision for the mentally ill, 82 ff.
Uranium, 19 f.

Vaccination, Army protected by, 8
Venereal disease, 10
Veterans, need for follow-up clinics, 65

Waksman, Selman A., 7
War, psychiatry and, 54 ff.; common neurotic reactions, 57 f.
Water, purification for drinking, 9
"What Has Psychiatry Learned during the Present War?" (Porter), 60*n*
Wolf, Katherine M., 44
Willow, extract, early use for rheumatic pains, 106

X-ray, use of, in medicine, 23 ff.; treatment for cancer, 30 ff.

Young, James, 52